BORN IN THE RIGHT BODY

Gender identity ideology from a medical and feminist perspective

Isidora Sanger

Copyright © 2022 by Dr Maja Bowen (writing as Isidora Sanger)

All rights reserved.

No part of this book may be reproduced in any form or by any electronic or mechanical means, including information storage and retrieval systems, without written permission from the author, except for the use of brief quotations in a book review.

Cover design by Al Peters@2cheeseburgers

❦ Created with Vellum

Contents

Foreword	v
1. About "Trans Women Are Women"	1
Bibliography	13
2. Conflation of Sex and Gender	17
Bibliography	23
3. What Is Sex?	25
Bibliography	33
4. There Is Nothing More Fundamental When Dealing With a Patient Than Knowing Whether They Are Male or Female	35
Bibliography	39
5. CASE STUDY 1 - Trans-identifying Female Being Evaluated for Kidney Transplant	41
Bibliography	47
6. Transgender Medicine as Departure From First Principles	49
Bibliography	69
7. Transactivist War on Reality - What They Think Studies Show vs What Studies Actually Show	71
Bibliography	83
8. The Impostor Fantasy	85
9. CASE STUDY 2 - Experiment of Induced Lactation in a Trans-identifying Male	91
Bibliography	101
10. It's Not "Woman" but "Transgender" That Is a Truly Elusive Term, And How This Relates to Statistics on Trans Youth Suicide	103
Bibliography	121
11. Why I Decided to Stop Using the Term "Trans Woman"	125

	Bibliography	135
12.	The Myth of "Virtuous Paedophile" and Why P Should Not Be a Part of LGBT+	137
	Bibliography	157
13.	CASE STUDY 3 - Deny, Attack, Reverse Victim and Offender (DARVO)	159
14.	Our Society Can't Function If It Can't Tell the Difference Between Fantasy and Reality	167
	Bibliography	187
15.	On Symbols and Totalitarianism	191
	Bibliography	199
16.	Letter to a Female Transactivist	201
17.	The Myth of Human Asexuality	209
	Bibliography	219
18.	On Intersex, Transgender and Women's Sport	221
	Bibliography	237
19.	How Did Medical Institutions Get Captured by Gender Identity Ideology?	241
	Bibliography	271
20.	CASE STUDY 4 - BMA Policy Capture	279
	Bibliography	293
21.	Examples of Gender Ideology in Medical Institutions	297
	Bibliography	331
22.	My Interview With FiLiA - A Feminist Doctor on Gender Identity Policies, Institutional Capture and Medicine (FiLiA, 2021)	339
	Bibliography	357
	Acknowledgments	361
	About the Author	363

Foreword

The essays in this book are intended both as stand-alone pieces and as pieces of a puzzle that will form a clear picture of how we, as a society, came to engage in biological sex denialism and callous disregard for women's sex-based rights.

I hope this book serves as a record of an ignoble moment in history that should not be swept under the carpet and forgotten.

Chapter 1

About "Trans Women Are Women"

For years, men who aspired to emulate women, whether by wearing stereotypically feminine make up and clothing or by undergoing medical gender reassignment, were referred to as "transwomen". More recently, however, the spelling was changed to "trans women". This enabled trans-activists to argue that "trans women are women" and, because women are adult human females, "trans women" must be female too.

When challenged, they say: "Yes we know sex is immutable, this is why trans women were always female, their sex was just wrongly assigned at birth. 'Trans' is just another descriptor for a woman - like 'tall woman', 'Black woman' or 'disabled woman'. There is no one way to be a woman. Some women have blonde hair, other women have a penis. This penis, by the virtue of belonging to a certain kind of 'woman', automatically becomes a 'female penis'. If you refuse to accept any of this, you are a trans-misogynistic bigot."

On the surface, this novel interpretation of the word "woman" may seem progressive and kind.

"If people tell you who they are - believe them. Acceptance without exception. Trans rights are human rights!"

The problem is, not only does the claim "trans women are women" have no basis in science or logic - men and women, males and females, are immutable biological sexes and circular definitions are meaningless - it also erases men who identify as women. Only men can be "trans women". This is evident from the fact that undergoing a process of "male-to-female transition" is a fundamental defining quality of being a "trans woman". Therefore, if you were never male to begin with, you were never a "trans woman" either.

This creation of a special category of "man", and simultaneous erasure of it in language, has had a profound effect on women, and on the men who wish to emulate them.

Medical implications

Historically, medical gender reassignment (formerly known as "sex change" or "sex reassignment") was designed to convert homosexual males into straight members of the opposite sex. These males suffered homophobic abuse throughout their lives, but instead of increasing tolerance toward them, society and the medical profession declared them "abnormal" and punished same-sex attraction. "Feminine essence", "man trapped in a woman's body", "born in the wrong body", "wrongly assigned male at birth" were all linguistic sleights of hand designed to obscure homophobia, as well as the fact some men feel so uncomfortable with their bodies and masculine social roles, they seek to drastically modify their appearance in order to escape them. If only his facial features were more feminine, voice higher, breasts larger, hair longer, then society would recognise him for the woman he really is on the inside, and he would feel happier.

This projection of psychological discomfort onto the body is not dissimilar to how some women feel so uncomfortable with their appearance and social roles, they starve themselves into losing secondary sexual characteristics and body fat. However, society generally agrees that it is harmful to affirm an anorexic's irrational belief that they are overweight and to offer liposuction as treatment for their distress. Why, then, is extreme body modification considered appropriate treatment for psychological distress at being born one sex and not the other?

Gender dysphoria, body dysmorphic disorder (BDD) and eating disorders are separate entities but in practice they often co-exist. A seemingly exclusive focus on body alteration as the desired intervention for those who identify as the opposite sex (which is practically synonymous with a psychiatric diagnosis of "gender dysphoria") means that body dysmorphia is a significant, if not dominant, trait in the transgender phenomenon.

Although BDD is a contraindication to cosmetic interventions - or at least considered to be a clinical presentation that requires careful multi-disciplinary team assessment - in practice, patients with BDD are under-diagnosed and can usually find a surgeon who is willing to operate, as long as the patient signs a consent form. Therefore, the practice of treating psychological discomfort with surgery, despite the likelihood of unsatisfactory outcomes, is not without a precedent.

However, "medical gender reassignment" goes beyond cosmetic procedures such as lip fillers and rhinoplasty. It involves removal of healthy body parts, such as double mastectomies and hysterectomies for women and castration and vaginoplasties for men, as well as an administration of opposite-sex hormones in doses high enough to masculinise females and feminise males. These interventions carry a high risk of medical injury such as debilitating post-operative complications, loss of function and a significant increase in long-term morbidity, mortality and suicide.

Considering that evidence shows the long-term mental health outcomes worsen post medical gender reassignment (Dhejne, et al., 2011), it is not clear what the rationale is for these interventions, or why trans-identifying patients are encouraged to risk their own health in pursuit of a costly, yet unattainable, goal of sex change.

Whether or not these patients resort to medication and surgery in order to "pass" as the opposite sex, society's conflation of self-declared "gender identity" with biological sex can also result in their biology being neglected in a clinical context (Dahlen, 2020; Wilson, 2021).

In the NHS, it has become common practice to change the sex markers on medical records to bring them in line with a patient's self-identified gender identity. (PCSE 2020)

This has created such confusion, that the NHS now invites men who changed their sex marker to "female" for smears of cervices they do not have, while not inviting them for sex-appropriate screening such as an ultrasound scan to check for the presence of abdominal aortic aneurysm. On the other hand, women who change their sex markers to "male" stop being automatically invited for sex-appropriate breast and cervical screening. Clinicians are expected to mitigate the risks of this, even though they report finding it increasingly difficult to bring up trans-identifying patients' biological sex in discussions about their health, lest they be accused of "misgendering" and "transphobia".

A further consequence of the mantra "trans women are women" specifically, is that men only need to state their pronouns are "she/her" and they are automatically placed on women's hospital and psychiatric wards (Helyar, Hill & Griffin, 2021). This system is not only completely open to abuse by male predators, it has also deprived women of much needed single-sex spaces at times when they are at their most vulnerable to male violence.

Social implications

Our society has long struggled to understand male violence against women. How can normally empathic men dehumanise women and treat them like things? How can they reduce the female half of the population to appearance and body parts, and fail to consider their humanity? The way men treat "trans women", as well as the way "trans women" reduce women to an objectified image held in the male gaze, can shed light on this issue.

Some of the loudest supporters of the idea that "trans women are women" are men who don't consider trans-identifying males as potential sexual partners, and if they are looking for a surrogate mother for their child, they are specifically looking for a biological female. Yet these men promote an ideology which holds that it is impossible, too complicated and hateful to answer the question "what is a woman" beyond saying "a woman is anyone who identifies as a woman".

On the other hand, lesbians are labelled as "bigots" for excluding trans-identifying men from their dating pool, and anyone who points out that "trans women" cannot be lesbians, because lesbians are same-sex attracted females and "trans women" are male, is denounced as a "transphobe".

This makes the mantra "trans women are women" just another tool with which men can oppress and coerce women.

Failing to acknowledge that "trans women" are men, also prevents us from understanding why other men feel the compulsion to exclude them from the sex class they naturally belong to. Instead of widening the bandwidth of what it means to "be a man", society has resorted to defining both women and "trans women" as "non-men", in an attempt to create an umbrella term for all those deemed lesser than the default, fully-fledged human beings.

In patriarchy, stereotypes of masculinity, and femininity, as well as the hierarchy between them, are considered "innate". If something is innate, a man doesn't need to feel bad for perpetrating it, and the misery of the victim as well as the benefit to the oppressor is just the natural order of things. Men have used these rationalisations to remain deaf to the plight of women for thousands of years, and they have punished anyone who has threatened the status quo - including men who break the masculinity code and willingly don the "uniform of the oppressed".

If wearing dresses and makeup, being submissive, gentle, nurturing and emotional aren't inherently female qualities, then maybe women's subjugated position in society isn't natural either?

Historically, men have inflicted violence on feminine men in order to resolve this cognitive dissonance. "You will either man up, cut your hair and put on the boring suit or you will get treated like a woman."

Whether "being treated as a woman" takes the form of physical violence and sexual assault or social exclusion and unethical medical interventions, it amounts to the kind of harm many women are familiar with.

Trans rights activism has thankfully raised awareness of this abusive dynamic, but it hasn't given feminine men the freedom to be who they truly are. Instead trans-identifying men are given the opportunity to police women from within the female sex class, which is a novel and particularly intrusive way of maintaining male supremacy.

"Trans women" are considered worthy of empathy and admiration for choosing to identify as the maligned (female) sex, while women and trans-identifying females (who supposedly acquired male privilege when they identified into the male sex class) are expected to give up their spaces and resources in order to accommodate "trans women" away from other males.

This mirrors existing inequality between the sexes. By allowing the desires of trans-identifying males to dominate discourse on both trans rights and women's rights, women's needs have become subjugated to men's wants. This is justified by assertions that this special category of males constitutes "the most oppressed minority in history", even though it is women who are still taking the brunt of gender discrimination and male violence.

Despite, or perhaps because of this, "trans women" are widely considered to be unwelcome intruders in women's spaces. They don't have female bodies, and because they are socialised as males, they retain male aggression and entitlement which makes many women feel unsafe. So they are excluded again, only this time, the basis for their exclusion is biology and the facts of life, not shunning by their own kind.

In order to obscure this, transactivists have attempted to dissociate female biology from the words "woman" and "female". The male half of humanity are now both "men" and "women", while the female half are split into "menstruators", "bleeders", "egg producers", "chest feeders", "vulva owners", "birthing bodies" and "people with vaginas". These "bodies" don't exist on a temporal continuum, going through different stages in life which include maturation, fertility, ageing and sex-specific diseases. They are nothing more than fragmented identities that some "people" might come to occupy, seemingly at random.

"Trans men are men. Their bodies have uteruses, cervices and ovaries. Therefore, men have periods, they can get pregnant and they also go through menopause. Men may need abortions too. Saying that woman is an adult human female is biological essentialism and therefore wrong. Woman is simply anyone who identifies as a woman, and 'trans women' definitely fit into that category."

Theft of the word "woman" from human females, in order to give it to some males, was made possible because of the existing social hierarchies. Trans-identifying females can neither endanger the rights, safety or social status of men, nor force men to accept them as "real men". The negative impact of gender self-identification on male privileges, such as primogeniture, was even legislated against in the Gender Recognition Act 2004, so an eldest daughter could not identify as male and take an inheritance and titles from her male siblings. (GRA, 2004)

No such provision was made for women. Instead, female-specific language, spaces and services were left open for any man to identify into and use as he sees fit.

Feminist implications

In 2015, the UK government held a first Trans Equality Enquiry, with a view to amending the Gender Recognition Act to allow gender self-identification.

Many women's groups opposed this, and professionals who work with sex offenders raised red flags.

For example, The British Psychological Society testified that psychologists who work with forensic patients are aware of a number of cases, where male sex offenders falsely claimed to be "transgender females". They did this: "a) As a means of demonstrating reduced risk and so gaining parole; b) As a means of explaining their sex offending aside from sexual gratification (e.g. wanting to 'examine' young females); c) Or as a means of separating their sex offending self (male) from their future self (female). d) In rare cases, it has been thought that the person is seeking better access to females and young children through presenting in an apparently female way."

They stated that instead of reducing risk, these strategies may increase it, and referred to the belief that males taking oestrogen and androgen blockers reduced their risk of offending, as "false". Therefore, while recommending that the Government give appropriate assistance to trans-identifying prisoners, they urged them to be "extremely cautious of setting law and policy such that some of the most dangerous people in society have greater latitude to offend." (Richards, 2015)

This sentiment was echoed by British Association of Gender Identity Specialists (BAGIS) who said that they were seeing "the ever-increasing tide of referrals of patients in prison serving long or indeterminate sentences for serious sexual offences. These vastly outnumber the number of prisoners incarcerated for more ordinary, non-sexual, offences."

They referred to suggestions that nobody would claim transsexual status in prison unless they really were transsexual, as "naive", and added that reasons to falsely claim transsexual status ranged from wanting special treatment, trips out of prison and transfer to the female estate (sometimes the same one as their female co-defendant), to seeking more favourable treatment at a parole hearing due to a belief that "a parole board will perceive somebody who is female as being less dangerous through a belief that hormone treatment will actually render one less dangerous".

They also warned that prison intelligence information indicated that the driving force behind male offenders claiming transsexual status might include a desire to make future sexual offending easier, because women are generally perceived to be low risk in this regard. (Barrett, 2015)

Investigating how even the most dangerous of men were allowed to self-identify as women and gain access to female single-sex facilities, revealed that transactivist organisations thought that allowing gender self-identification in the most extreme and risky scenario would make it easier to embed this practice in other contexts.

As James Morton, the Manager of Scottish Trans Alliance, explained: "Another key priority was pushing for public services to always respect trans people's gender identities, even if they have not changed all their official documents or attended an NHS gender identity clinic. We strategised that by working intensively with the Scottish Prison Service to support them to include trans women as women on a self-declaration basis within very challenging circumstances, we would be able to ensure that all other public services should be able to do likewise." (Burns, 2018; FWS, 2021)

The Twitter thread that inspired this essay was written in 2018, when most of us were just starting to discover the full impact that the mantra "transwomen are women" was having on the safety of women and children. Since then, we have learned it has become mandatory to affirm the self-declared "female gender identity" of male criminals, even though over half of transgender prisoners in England and Wales are sex offenders, and the nature of their offences suggests that the vast majority are men (FPFW, 2017).

The Judicial Review brought on by a female inmate who was raped by one such man, ruled that the practice of putting these men in female prisons was "lawful" (WPUK, 2021), and now, female inmates who raise concerns about this, or refuse to address these men using "she/her" pronouns, risk being punished and even having time added to their sentences (Inside Time, 2021).

Thanks to the influence of transactivists on the Equal Treatment Bench Book (Chacko, 2021), women assaulted by trans-identifying men have already been compelled in court to refer to their male attackers as "she" (Moss, 2018), while employees of Family Court report that men who declare a "female gender identity" are circumventing safeguarding checks by having their previous name and biological sex deleted from the records (la scapigliata, 2021).

Similar institutional policies have allowed men to not only gain access to women's hospital wards (Dixon, 2021), rape crisis services (FWS, 2021), domestic violence shelters (McDonald, 2022), toilets, changing rooms (Hosie, 2018), sports (Aschwanden, 2019) and women-only shortlists (BBC, 2018), but they have done so despite knowing this would lead women to self-exclude from essential services.

None of this serves to increase acceptance. If anything, the mantra "trans women are women" has brought about outcomes that cast suspicion on all such men, and despite the temporary power grab, it has reinforced the societal impression that they have ulterior motives.

More widely, and by their very nature, ideologies that assert the supremacy of personal choice in an unequal and inequitable society often legitimise terrible outcomes for the most vulnerable. They ignore the reality that certain demographics hold power over others and that those who are truly oppressed can never identify out of their oppression, nor do they have the level of freedom necessary to really choose. Examples of some of the harms previously legitimised by "choice" ideologies include pornography, prostitution, commercial surrogacy and forced labour.

Eager to change policies "in advance of the law", UK political parties are allowing candidates to self-identify as women, disabled or ethnic minorities, while we are led to believe that by erasing all meaningful social categories, they are ushering in a new age where discrimination will become a thing of the past.

Why, then, are able-bodied, white men still, overwhelmingly, in charge?

Why are councils painting rainbows and trans-flags on pedestrian crossings, despite numerous complaints that they are frightening police horses and guide dogs and confusing people with sensory processing disabilities? (Gant, 2021)

Why are women - who are still being exploited, raped and murdered by men at no reduced rate - still being painted as villains when they say No to "trans women" in women's spaces? Especially when statistics show that these men are more likely to be perpetrators than victims of homicide (Trans Crime UK, 2017)?

I fear that the practice of gender self-identification, which includes the mantra "trans women are women", rather than being a grassroots movement for justice and liberation, only serves to perpetuate abusive gender dynamics.

That our society was so widely captured by this ideology, is the issue I have explored in depth in the following essays.

Bibliography

Dhejne, C. Lichtenstein, P. Boman, M. Johansson, A. L. V. Långström, N. et al. (2011) Long-Term Follow-Up of Transsexual Persons Undergoing Sex Reassignment Surgery: Cohort Study in Sweden. PLOS ONE 6(2): e16885. https://doi.org/10.1371/journal.pone.0016885

Dahlen, S. (2020) De-sexing the Medical Record? An Examination of Sex Versus Gender Identity in the General Medical Council's Trans Healthcare Ethical Advice. The New Bioethics. 26:1. 38-52. https://www.tandfonline.com/doi/full/10.1080/20502877.2020.1720429

Wilson, C. (2021). NHS patient 'self identification' risking healthcare study warns. HeraldScotland. https://www.heraldscotland.com/news/19207717.nhs-self-identification-policy-risking-patients-healthcare-study-warns/

PCSE. (2020). Process for registering a patient gender re-assignment. Pcse.england.nhs.uk. https://pcse.england.nhs.uk/media/1291/process-for-registering-a-patient-gender-re-assignment.pdf

Helyar, S. Hill, A. Griffin, L. (2021). Nurses request that health and nursing organisations withdraw from Stonewall's Diversity Championship Scheme. https://lascapigliata.com/institutional-capture/nurses-request-that-health-and-nursing-organisations-withdraw-from-stonewalls-diversity-championship-scheme/

GRA 2004. Explanatory notes 80. https://www.legislation.gov.uk/ukpga/2004/7/notes/division/4/16

Richards, C. (2015). Written evidence - The British Psychological Society. Data.parliament.uk. http://data.parliament.uk/WrittenEvidence/CommitteeEvidence.svc/EvidenceDocument/Women%20and%20Equalities/Transgender%20Equality/written/19471.html

Barrett, J. (2015). Written evidence - British Association Of Gender Identity Specialists. Data.parliament.uk. http://data.parliament.uk/WrittenEvidence/CommitteeEvidence.svc/EvidenceDocument/Women%20and%20Equalities/Transgender%20Equality/written/19532.html

Burns, C. (2018). Trans Britain: Our Journey from the Shadows. Unbound (25 Jan. 2018). Chapter 12, page 240.

FWS. (2021). The Status of Women In Scotland – Prisons. For Women Scotland. https://forwomen.scot/03/08/2021/the-status-of-women-in-scotland-prisons/

FPFW (2017). Half of all transgender prisoners are sex offenders or dangerous category A inmates. Fair Play For Women. https://fairplayforwomen.com/transgender-prisoners/

WPUK. (2021). Women's prisons and male transgender prisoners. Woman's Place UK. https://womansplaceuk.org/2021/07/07/womens-prisons-male-transgender-prisoners/

Inside Time. (2021). Women face punishment for using wrong pronouns. https://insidetime.org/women-face-punishment-for-using-wrong-pronouns/

Chacko, T. (2021). Prejudging the transgender controversy? Why the Equal Treatment Bench Book needs urgent revision. Policyexchange.org.uk. https://policyexchange.org.uk/wp-content/uploads/2021/07/Prejudging-the-transgender-controversy-.pdf

Moss, J. (2021). INTERVIEW: Maria MacLachlan on the GRA and the aftermath of her assault at Speaker's Corner. Feminist Current. https://www.feministcurrent.com/2018/06/21/interview-maria-maclauchlan-gra-aftermath-assault-speakers-corner/

la scapigliata. (2021). Family court employee. https://lascapigliata.com/institutional-capture/family-court-employee/

Dixon, H. (2021). Patient safety fears as NHS allows trans sex offenders in female-only wards. https://www.telegraph.co.uk/news/2021/08/02/safety-fears-patients-nhs-allows-trans-sex-offenders-female/

FWS. (2021). The Real Crisis at Rape Crisis Scotland - For Women Scotland. https://forwomen.scot/10/08/2021/the-real-crisis-at-rape-crisis-scotland/

McDonald, H. (2022). Transgender paedophile, who was born a man but identifies as female, is caught duping staff for 71-day stay at domestic violence refuge centre for vulnerable women. https://www.dailymail.co.uk/news/article-11392601/Transgender-paedophile-caught-duping-staff-71-day-stay-domestic-violence-refuge.html

Hosie, R. (2018). Unisex changing rooms put women at danger of sexual assault, data reveals. The Independent. https://www.independent.co.uk/life-style/women/sexual-assault-unisex-changing-rooms-sunday-times-women-risk-a8519086.html

Aschwanden, C. (2019). Trans Athletes Are Posting Victories and Shaking Up Sports. https://www.wired.com/story/the-glorious-victories-of-trans-athletes-are-shaking-up-sports/

BBC. (2018). Labour: Row over inclusion of trans women in all-women shortlists. https://www.bbc.co.uk/news/uk-politics-43962349

Gant, J. (2021). Virtue-signalling councils ditch zebra crossings: Camden is latest authority to unveil trans-friendly path despite safety warning after police horse is spooked by LGBT rainbow and guide dog is baffled by missing white lines. https://www.dailymail.co.uk/news/article-10181979/Camden-trans-walkway-New-zebra-crossing-causes-chaos-guide-dog-police-horse.html

Trans Crime UK. (2017). Trans homicides in the UK: a closer look at the numbers. http://transcrimeuk.com/2017/11/16/trans-homicides-in-the-uk-a-closer-look-at-the-numbers/

Chapter 2

Conflation of Sex and Gender

For most people, the first association they make when they hear the word 'sex' is "sexual intercourse". 'Sex' is a word that is simultaneously taboo and central to our culture. Sex sells products in advertising, and selling sex is a product in itself. So much of human culture revolves around discussing sex, wanting it, controlling it, envying and shaming those who have it and pitying and idealising those who do not. Sex - or intercourse - is a source of neurosis in all of human culture, including the Christian West, which has made a virtue out of celibacy and the repression of sexual urges thus contributing to a society-wide obsession with it.

However, 'sex' is a homonym - a word with two meanings - and apart from sexual intercourse it also refers to biological categories involved in sexual reproduction.

Humans, like all other sexually reproducing organisms, can be divided into males and females. Men and boys constitute the male sex and women and girls constitute the female sex.

Due to our collective discomfort with the topic of sexual

intercourse, 'gender' has become a polite euphemism for biological sex. However, 'gender' also refers to the social stereotypes of appearance and behaviour imposed on people depending on their biological sex. Males are supposed to be "masculine" and females are supposed to be "feminine" in both appearance and behaviour, and to make matters even more complicated, 'gender' is also a grammatical term.

In the English language, pronouns are sex-based. A female person or animal - such as 'girl' or 'hen' - is referred to as "she/her/hers", while 'boy' or 'rooster' is referred to as "he/him/his". Generic nouns used to denote juvenile animals or inanimate objects, such as 'lamb' or 'table', are referred to by the 'gender-neutral' pronouns "it/its".

In gendered languages, such as Latin, while nouns that refer to females are feminine - such as 'puella, puellae [f.]' (girl) - and nouns that refer to males are masculine - such as 'puer, pueri [m.]' (boy) - grammatical gender is mostly arbitrary, that is to say that masculinity of a noun does not imply maleness and vice versa.

For example, in Latin, 'uterus, uteri [m.]' (womb) is a masculine noun, and in French, 'le chat' (cat) is masculine, while 'la fraternité' (brotherhood) is feminine. The Romans didn't labour under the delusion that uteruses are male reproductive organs, nor do the French believe all cats are male, or that men organising into brotherhoods makes them "female". Instead it is simply a grammatical quality that influences the word endings (declensions), pronouns and adjectives, which accompany different nouns.

Therefore, I was puzzled to see 'gender' used instead of 'sex' throughout the English literature, scientific or otherwise. This convention doesn't make sense in languages that have gendered nouns, and you can see discussions about this on many translator forums. Seeing a native English speaker trying to explain the socio-cultural meaning of the word 'gender' to, say, a native French speaker, inevitably involves a lot of postmodernist ideas such as "denaturalising gender performance" and "gender being an arbitrary cultural concept" which nonetheless applies to males and females differently with regards to the gendered norms of appearance and behaviour.

However confident English speakers might be that they indeed appreciate the nuance between sex and gender, the interchangeable way in which they use "female gender" and "feminine gender" tells a different story.

It is not clear when 'gender' was first used as a polite euphemism for biological sex, but it seems to have been popularised by the sexologist John Money in the 1960s (Goldie, 2014). Money initially defined 'gender' based on the sex differences between human beings. Females are smaller, they produce ova and bear young while males are bigger, they produce sperm and impregnate females. As a believer in the idea that our internal sense of whether we are male or female stems not from our sexed bodies but from the way we are socialised from infancy, Money went beyond human sexual dimorphism and "sex roles" to coin the phrase "gender roles", which denotes the socially constructed stereotypes of masculinity and femininity.

These stereotypes are opposing qualities that change across time and cultures, but their purpose is always to create a social hierarchy in which members of the male sex class are privileged over members of the female sex class. This hierarchy is then justified by the idea that males are naturally dominant, active, logical, decisive and worldly, while females are naturally submissive, passive, emotional, indecisive and home-oriented. These prescribed standards of behaviour remain deeply embedded in our culture despite evidence that most humans don't fit neatly into these gendered boxes.

This is quite different from the sex categories of 'male' and 'female' which apply to all humans without exception.

Almost all humans are normally sexed, and those who are born with disorders of sex development (DSDs) are still either male or female, albeit with some differences from the norm. Because humans are a sexually dimorphic species, our biological sex is readily apparent, and in the rare cases where it is not, it is easily determined by physical examination, imaging and genetic testing. Therefore, sex has a certain finality about it – it is factually observable, confirmed throughout nature and it is integral to the way we function and reproduce. Whether our sex is male or female is not a value judgement in and of itself, until gender is superimposed onto it.

An effeminate, passive, caring male or an assertive, dominant, masculine female are only perceived as gender non-conforming, transgressive or even "problematic" when their personality, style, physical appearance and interests challenge gender stereotypes which underpin the gender hierarchy.

By imposing gender stereotypes on humans from birth, an unequal society is created where stereotypes of masculinity are conflated with the male sex and femininity is conflated with the female sex, in order to claim males are naturally superior and females naturally inferior. Men and boys are taught to be entitled to women and girls' physical, emotional and domestic labour, while women and girls are taught to take care of, prioritise and appease males. This is the bedrock of patriarchy, and the reason why gender is both inherently discriminatory to the female sex, and why males and females who resist these socially imposed gender roles are deemed "abnormal" and discriminated against.

How does discrimination justify itself? By claiming that it's natural.

We have seen both racial and gender stereotypes defended as natural before, and anything from bias in research and misinterpretation of evidence to filtering findings through the lens of ideology and a censorship of opposing views, is used to legitimise the status quo. Furthermore, by hijacking words that mean 'sex' (man, woman, boy, girl, male, female) and using them as synonyms for words that mean 'gender' (masculine, feminine), gender has exploited the factual validity associated with sex in order to legitimise itself.

Cue the term 'cis' - an archaic term which means "on this side of" - which in the language of gender ideology means that a person identifies with gender stereotypes imposed on their sex. Likewise, the term 'trans' - which means "on the opposite side of" - is repurposed by gender ideology to mean that a person identifies with gender stereotypes imposed on the opposite sex.

'Cis' and 'trans' have been used to reduce women to a subset of their own sex class ("cis women"), which now also includes males ("trans women").

If a man is perceived as feminine, then he must really be a "woman". 'Trans' is just an adjective in this scenario and therefore, "trans women are women, just like tall women, Black women or indeed cis women".

Furthermore, because males are socialised to dominate females, "trans women" are considered to be a superior kind of woman and deferred to on all issues pertaining to the female sex.

This is how we got to the point where women who speak about the biological reality of living in a female body, and the negative impact of males in female-only spaces, are called "transphobes", "TERFS" and "exclusionary bigots", while the men who reduce the female sex to gender stereotypes so they can embody them and gain access to spaces and services reserved for females, are posited as "victims" of women's boundaries.

Although convoluted and language-specific, the tactic of conflating sex and gender has been so successful that 'gender' is now replacing 'sex' in law and policy all over the world, thereby obliterating the sex-based protections that women and girls need in order to mitigate the effects of male violence.

This cautionary tale is a good example of how imperfect language is, and how it can be weaponised to redefine reality and laws for a specific agenda. For this reason, whenever new definitions of common words appear out of nowhere and new laws are being proposed based on poorly defined terms, the best way to avoid pitfalls is to examine them critically and ask: What impact will this have in the real world?

Bibliography

Goldie, T. (2014). The Man Who Invented Gender: Engaging the Ideas of John Money. Ubcpress.ca. https://www.ubcpress.ca/asset/9338/1/9780774827928.pdf

Chapter 3

What Is Sex?

Biological sex is a fundamental differentiating factor between two types of bodies required for a species to reproduce sexually. In humans, a baby who is born with a vagina, uterus and ovaries typically produces ova and has 46 XX chromosomes, while a baby who is born with a penis and testicles typically produces sperm and has 46 XY chromosomes. (Gilbert SF, 2000)

The vast majority of humans are born with normal sex characteristics. This situation is so overwhelmingly consistent that just by observing external genitalia at birth doctors, midwives and parents can be certain that in almost all cases they will be right in calling a baby a boy or a girl. This is also true in cases of common genital abnormalities, such as hypospadias. This relatively common condition, which results in a urethral opening not being located in its usual position at the tip of the penis, doesn't cause any ambiguity because affected boys still have the characteristics which are fully consistent with the male sex. (Sax, 2002)

In their quest to justify normally sexed people self-identifying as the opposite sex, transactivists have used the very small percentage of people with Disorders of Sex Development (DSDs, previously termed "intersex") to claim that "sex is a spectrum" and that identifying as the opposite sex is some kind of "intersex condition of the brain". To this end, they quote obscure brain imaging studies which claim to have found evidence that males can have a "female brain" and vice versa.

I will critically appraise one of these studies in a later essay, but suffice it to say, the only way for a brain to be female is for it to exist inside a female body. Sex in humans can't be changed and, while there are many misconceptions surrounding DSDs, including their repeated conflation with transgenderism, there is no evidence that people who identify as the opposite sex have a higher incidence of abnormal sex development than the general population (Pang et al, 2018; Inoubli et al, 2011).

What is true is that despite atypical features, people with DSDs have a biological sex, and over the years medicine has explored different ways to determine and define sex in this specific context. Medicine has also unsuccessfully engaged in attempts to change the biological sex of people with DSDs as well as adult homosexuals and crossdressers, which has given rise to the controversial practice of "sex change".

Since the early 20th century, doctors have conducted experiments to see if it was possible to change a man into a woman - and vice versa. The methods were almost identical to those used today - patients were asked to present socially as the opposite sex, and males were "feminised" while females were "masculinised" with opposite sex hormones and cosmetic and genital surgeries.

This practice didn't enter into the medical mainstream until Johns Hopkins hospital, in Baltimore, started offering these experimental procedures in 1965. One of the key figures involved in this area of medicine was a psychotherapist and sexologist called John Money. He believed that "gender identity" - or our internal sense of whether we are male or female - is malleable and could be socially constructed. To this end, he had already been working with Claude Migeon, to "reassign" the sex of children who were born with ambiguous genitalia.

During his long and controversial career, John Money coined the terms "gender role", "sexual orientation" and "paraphilia", and following his studies on "hermaphrodites" he identified six variables that defined sex, whilst acknowledging that in most people all six will align.

It's worth mentioning that "hermaphrodite", just like "intersex", when applied to humans is a misnomer. For a human to be a hermaphrodite, they would either need to have fully functioning male *and* female reproductive organs or to be able to change sex and be fertile as males and females at different points during their lifetime. There are no known cases of this ever occurring in humans, or indeed mammals. As medicine gained further understanding, the terminology changed to "pseudo-hermaphroditism", DSDs (disorders/differences of sex development) and VSDs (variations in sex development).

DSD advocates have long asked both transactivists and the medical profession to stop using terms such as "intersex" and "hermaphrodite" to describe them, as these terms are erroneous and stigmatising. Unfortunately, these misnomers still persist in some areas of medical literature, and they have been resurrected with enthusiasm by those who seek to misappropriate DSD terminology for the purposes of transactivism.

One of John Money's most famous, and tragic, cases involved a Canadian boy called David Reimer and his twin brother Brian. When David was a baby, he suffered extensive injuries to his penis following a botched circumcision. Concerned about their son's future happiness, his parents took him to see John Money at Johns Hopkins Hospital in 1967. They were persuaded by Money, and his medical team, that their son would be happier if he was raised as a girl. David Reimer's sex was "reassigned" at 22 months - his testes were removed and a rudimentary vulva fashioned in place of the injured penis - and he and his brother continued to see John Money throughout their childhood and adolescence. In order to "solidify" a female gender identity, Money forced the Reimer twins to simulate sexual play, with David in the "female role". These sessions were ostensibly designed to convince David that he was female, however, on at least one occasion, Money is said to have taken naked photographs of the boys. Considering that John Money also claimed that non-sadistic paedophilia was an "excess of parental love" and therefore "not pathological", it is not surprising that the Reimer twins ended up severely traumatised by these experiences. David is said to have realised he was in fact a boy between the ages of nine and eleven. By thirteen, he developed a suicidal depression and refused to see Money again. By fifteen, he started living his life as a male.

Unfortunately, the Reimer twins never fully recovered from their ordeal. They both suffered great disruption to their lives and struggled with mental health issues. As a consequence, Brian died of a drug overdose in 2002, and David committed suicide in 2004. (Gaetano, 2017)

I remember sitting in the lecture theatre in 1998, a year after David Reimer first publicly spoke out about the medical abuse he and his brother had suffered. The room was quiet apart from the strangled voice of the lecturer, who told us about the horrific medical scandal that had been perpetrated by Money, and other doctors, who had also experimented on children with abnormal genitalia. Remembering that just a couple of years earlier, another professor was almost giddy with excitement when he hypothesised that humans can indeed have an opposite sex brain in their own bodies, a chill ran straight through me. For decades John Money claimed the Reimer experiment was a success and his belief that gender identity could be socially constructed was accepted by the medical mainstream, leading to thousands of abusive procedures being carried out not only on DSD children but also on physically healthy gender non-conforming adults.

This occurred despite the fact Johns Hopkins Hospital stopped offering gender reassignment procedures in 1979, amid concerns. They stated that these interventions carried significant risks while offering no objective benefit in terms of social rehabilitation. They came to this conclusion by comparing patients who received these procedures with patients who sought "sex reassignment" but remained unoperated on at follow-up (Pauly, 1981; Meyer & Reter, 1979).

After this, "sex change" experiments on gender non-conforming adults still continued to be performed on the margins of the medical profession, until eventually, this practice experienced a renaissance in the context of the transgender movement, which successfully shifted the narrative from "sex change" to "gender reassignment" and eventually "gender affirmation".

The problem today is the same as it ever was. Sex in humans is determined at conception, by the presence or absence of the Y chromosome, and it remains immutable ever after. Doctors have never made a man's penis and testicles change into a vagina, uterus and ovaries, nor vice versa, and our sex chromosomes likewise cannot be changed. The latter is the most important because, apart from directing the development of the foetus in utero, gene expression differs between males and females and sex differences consequently reside in every cell of our body.

This has wide-ranging consequences on form and function. (Deegan & Engel, 2019)

Sex reassignment has only ever gone as far as cosmetically altering the body to superficially resemble the opposite sex and this includes the creation of "neo-genitals" which look somewhat similar to real genitals but are constructed artificially, and are therefore unable to replicate the function of natural sex organs.

While some people with DSDs also undergo surgeries to create neo-genitals, these operations are carried out to treat medical problems which arise from congenital abnormalities. This is quite different from removing the healthy body parts of people who identify as the opposite sex, and replacing them with surgical simulacrums. Particularly given this is done in the pursuit of the idea that, where our perception of the body is at odds with reality, it is the body that needs to be changed to bring it in line with the disordered mind.

Neo-genitals are functional for intercourse purposes alone. They have to be manually dilated, lubricated, pumped into erection and managed by the patient for the rest of their lives. Natural genitals, in contrast, autonomously perform a multitude of functions, from intercourse, urination and ejaculation to menstruation and acting as birth canals.

Even if a trans-identifying patient is prepared to post-operatively manage their neo-genitals there are long-term risks associated with these operations, as well as the rest of the gender reassignment treatment pathway. Puberty blockers followed by the long-term usage of cross-sex hormones not only increase the likelihood of surgical complications - because in the absence of puberty, a penis never fully develops and surgeries to create neo-genitals are thus more complex and prone to failure - they also increase the risk of impaired bone and brain development and cardiovascular disease.

The take home message here is: it is important to keep in mind that biological sex cannot be changed by any known medical procedure. Additionally, while rare abnormalities of sex development do exist, they neither explain the psychological phenomenon of opposite sex identification, nor do they redefine the male and female sex categories.

Bibliography

Gilbert SF. (2000). Chromosomal Sex Determination in Mammals. Developmental Biology. 6th edition. Sunderland (MA): Sinauer Associates. https://www.ncbi.nlm.nih.gov/books/NBK9967/

Sax L. (2002). How common is intersex? a response to Anne Fausto-Sterling. Journal of sex research, 39(3), 174–178. https://www.leonardsax.com/how-common-is-intersex-a-response-to-anne-fausto-sterling/

Pang, K. C. Feldman, D. Oertel, R. Telfer, M. (2018). Molecular Karyotyping in Children and Adolescents with Gender Dysphoria. Transgender Health, Dec 2018, 147-153. http://doi.org/10.1089/trgh.2017.0051

Inoubli, A. De Cuypere, G. Rubens, R. Heylens, G. Elaut, E. Van Caenegem, E. Menten, B. & T'Sjoen, G. (2011). Karyotyping, is it worthwhile in transsexualism?. The journal of sexual medicine, 8(2), 475–478. https://doi.org/10.1111/j.1743-6109.2010.02130.x

Gaetano, P. (2017). David Reimer and John Money Gender Reassignment Controversy: The John/Joan Case. Embryo Project Encyclopedia (2017-11-15). ISSN: 1940-5030. http://embryo.asu.edu/handle/10776/13009

Pauly I. B. (1981). Outcome of sex reassignment surgery for transsexuals. The Australian and New Zealand journal of psychiatry, 15(1), 45–51. https://doi.org/10.3109/00048678109159409

Meyer, J. K., & Reter, D. J. (1979). Sex reassignment. Follow-up. Archives of general psychiatry, 36(9), 1010–1015. https://doi.org/10.1001/archpsyc.1979.01780090096010

Deegan, D.F. Engel, N. (2019). Sexual Dimorphism in the Age of Genomics: How, When, Where. Front. Cell Dev. Biol., 06 September 2019. https://doi.org/10.3389/fcell.2019.00186

Chapter 4

There Is Nothing More Fundamental When Dealing With a Patient Than Knowing Whether They Are Male or Female

Humans can't change their biological sex, but thanks to the practice of "medical gender reassignment" they can appear like the opposite sex. In the past - before puberty blocking followed by cross-sex hormones became the mainstay in managing childhood gender dysphoria - gender-reassigned patients, or transsexuals, were both rare and more easily recognisable as members of their own sex class. Now, a male-looking teen presenting with abdominal pain could in fact be a pregnant female who is, or was, taking masculinising doses of testosterone. A broken arm could be a consequence of bone thinning due to puberty blockers. The risk of blood clots is increased in both males and females who are on cross-sex hormone treatment. This is relevant to someone presenting with sudden onset chest pain or cough. Even some medications that are routinely given to sick patients are known to interact with exogenous sex hormones. To come back to the male-identifying female adolescent, there is another concern; if she presented with a broken arm it would be essential to know her pregnancy status before sending her off for a diagnostic x-ray.

Being male or female makes certain diagnoses, complications, prognoses, effects and side-effects of treatments more or less likely. Normal blood test values vary between the sexes and not knowing the true sex of a patient could lead to under treatment, over treatment, missing a diagnosis or making a wrong one. This also affects cancer screening. As mentioned previously, trans-identifying patients with opposite sex markers on their medical records are receiving invitations for wrong-sex cancer screening. The medical institutions seem to be leaving it up to individual patients to inform clinicians whether they are male or female, even though we are told that trans-identifying people find any mention of their biological sex "invalidating" and "offensive".

This no longer only affects trans-identifying patients. Thanks to gender self-identification policies, female patients can no longer be reassured that they have access to single-sex facilities and same-sex clinicians. Blood donation services are categorising blood products according to self-identified gender instead of biological sex. Considering that certain blood products from women who have been pregnant may increase the risk of transfusion reactions, especially in male recipients, allowing gender-identity ideology to influence healthcare policy risks a potential increase in adverse events for an ever increasing pool of patients.

The ideological capture has escalated so much now that doctors and nurses risk being shamed on social media for even asking whether a patient is transgender, which transactivists consider to be "bigotry akin to racism", while medical institutions are rushing to apologise to offended activists and to discipline clinicians. This cannot continue.

Transgenderism is a phenomenon closely associated with physical illness. When we decide to masculinise females and feminise males, we induce iatrogenic (treatment-caused) medical conditions. Puberty blockers, for example, decrease bone density causing spinal fractures and pain in gender dysphoric children (SVT, 2021), while flooding female bodies with enough testosterone to cause balding, deepening of the voice and uterine atrophy, or male bodies with enough oestrogen to induce breast development, induces endocrine disorders in both.

Anyone who has a chronic medical condition knows they'll be thoroughly quizzed about it every time they have a new presenting complaint, or are seeing a new doctor. This is not discriminatory, it is best medical practice.

To many marginalised groups certain questions by doctors can seem discriminatory and intrusive but there is a very good reason these questions are being asked. HIV status, Hep B and C are not uncommon, for example, but having tattoos is more of a Hep C risk factor if obtained in prison than in a tattoo parlour. A past history of somatic delusions, when combined with negative results from repeated investigations, informs our approach to presenting complaints.

It's impossible to fully convey to a layperson just how intricately medical history, examination and treatment are connected but it is important for everyone to understand that there is no clinical context where full history taking isn't essential. The sex of the patient, or if they are or ever were trans (and how far into transition they went ie. whether they took medications, which ones, for how long and whether they had gender-affirming surgery) is always relevant.

Transactivists can't have it both ways – demand medicalisation for trans-identifying people and force doctors to ignore it, under some misguided notion that mentioning biology in a healthcare context is "inappropriate". That this has become orthodoxy in medicine is a sign that political activists have been given ideological control over health professionals, without having any expertise or responsibility for the subsequent clinical outcomes.

Bibliography

SVT. (2021). Uppdrag granskning (Trans Train Pt IV). Mission: Investigate: Trans children. https://www.svtplay.se/video/33358590/uppdrag-granskning/mission-investigate-trans-children-avsnitt-1?id=jp9dBRA

Chapter 5

CASE STUDY 1 - Trans-identifying Female Being Evaluated for Kidney Transplant

In 2017, the Clinical Chemistry journal published a case study (Whitley & Greene, 2017) about a 33 year old trans-identifying woman who presented to the Emergency Department with an acute ear infection and high blood pressure. Her medication regime included daily atorvastatin and intramuscular testosterone cypionate injections (100 mg/week).

The patient refused admission, citing concerns that she would be discriminated against as a "transgender man", but she agreed to attend her GP surgery the following morning. The investigations revealed elevated protein in her urine, and her glomerular filtration rate (eGFR) - which is an indication of kidney function - was estimated to be 31 mL/min/1.73m2 if assessed using the male equation or 23 mL/min/1.73m2 if assessed using the female equation. She was diagnosed with stage 3 chronic kidney disease, prescribed a beta blocker to treat her high blood pressure and encouraged to stop testosterone as it could be adversely affecting her kidney function.

The patient agreed to follow this treatment plan, but then

she transferred to an alternate institution where testosterone injections were re-started, she was prescribed an ACE inhibitor and encouraged to reduce salt and protein in her diet, even though she had been a vegan for over 10 years.

Several months later, she was assessed for a kidney transplant using male equations again, which estimated her eGFR to be 23 mL/min/1.73m2.

Many variables affect kidney function values, from sex-specific differences to muscle mass, age, ethnicity, medications and diet. Masculinising doses of testosterone, for example, can disturb haemoglobin and haematocrit values in women to resemble that of men, while kidney function tends to remain sex-typical (Roberts et al 2014). This is why trans-identified patients often need additional investigations in order for the medical team to make an accurate assessment. These patients rely on the medical team to think laterally, rather than put ideology, and a patient's need for validation of their opposite-sex identity, at the centre of their healthcare plan.

In this case, the patient met most of the criteria for kidney transplant, such as the physical and psychological assessment which showed she would be able to adhere to the post-transplant regimen. The only criterion she didn't meet was the eGFR <20. Had the medical team not lost sight of the fact that sex cannot be changed, instead of using male equations to assess a female patient's kidney function they would have used female equations. In which case her eGFR would have been 18 mL/min/1.73m2 and she would have qualified for the kidney transplant.

Considering that the patient's body habitus (small, low muscle mass) was similar to the average woman, it beggars belief that her biological sex was repeatedly ignored when the stakes were so high. Also, it remains unclear whether the implications of continuing with testosterone injections were discussed with her.

Whitley & Greene tell us that "the patient's kidney disease etiology was unrelated to his transgender identity, it was attributed to him having Kawasaki's disease as a toddler". However, I am not sure that can be so definitively claimed since increases in testosterone have a known association with deteriorating kidney function (Filler et al 2016).

This female patient continued to experience suboptimal medical care due to her medical team treating her as if she was a biological male. A year after she first presented she demanded to be approved for the kidney transplant but she was met with resistance because her "male" eGFR was still greater than 20. Only when her "male" eGFR dropped to 18 was she finally put on a transplant list.

The medical team's continuing insistence on using male equations also complicated the issues around dialysis, causing delays and a suboptimal treatment regime. The fact that by the time dialysis was initiated she weighed only 100 lb, compared to 135 lb at her initial presentation, is a damning illustration of her body's decline. That this could have been possibly prevented by doctors adhering to what they knew to be true all along - that humans can't change sex – is alarming.

I would like to thank Whitley & Greene for bringing this important case to the attention of the wider medical community. However, I am concerned about their continuous use of male pronouns to describe a female patient. While I agree that doctors should be mindful about the intersection of transgenderism and medicine, accurate communication in a clinical context is absolutely essential. Medical staff consistently using wrong-sex pronouns when discussing patients' treatment plans, or ordering investigations, can negatively impact decision-making and result in clinical errors. The solution is not to continue using wrong sex pronouns and walking on eggshells around transgender patients. We are treating biological beings, whose sex is immutable. While we should always keep patient preferences in mind, we must not allow ideology or politics to override sound clinical judgement.

Had transgender ideology not been allowed to obfuscate the most fundamental reality about patients – that they are all members of a sexually dimorphic species and that sexual dimorphism profoundly affects their medical treatment (Horvath, 2021) - this patient would've been flagged up as a trans-identified female on cross-sex hormones. Her medical team would've been ethically compelled to keep her biological sex in mind at all times, and they would've been able to see her more clearly for who she was as a whole person rather than the collection of gender stereotypes that constitute transgender identity.

Nobody is born in the wrong body. The "sexed soul" doesn't just knock on the wrong door at conception and, even if it did, doctors would have a responsibility to treat the body, not neglect it. We've been fighting ideologies in order to protect vulnerable patients throughout the history of medicine. How is our responsibility to give a life-saving blood transfusion to a child of a Jehovah's Witness any different from our responsibility to avoid unnecessary delays in kidney transplants for a trans-identifying patient?

In the commentary following this article, Dr Greg Miller pointed out that:

"Using an estimated GFR when the patient does not represent an 'average' individual is not appropriate. It should have been obvious that a person who is 5 feet 1 inch in height, 100 pounds in weight, and is of slight build is not an 'average' individual for whom an estimate of GFR from creatinine would be suitable for use. This limitation would be correct irrespective of the actual gender, but the estimate for a biological female is more likely to be correct in this case. In addition, the NKDEP website specifically states that estimated GFR based on creatinine is not suitable for people eating either a vegetarian or a low-meat diet, as was the patient in this case." (Miller, 2017)

Dr Miller gives a very welcome clarification that should help clinicians avoid repeating such a mistake in the future. However, gender identity ideology has already demonstrated the power to compel clinicians to ignore what their own eyes, instincts and years of clinical experience are trying to tell them. Therefore, I fear that as long as this ideology is allowed to unduly influence medical practice all patient care will be compromised.

Bibliography

Whitley, C. Greene, D. (2017) Transgender Man Being Evaluated for a Kidney Transplant. Clinical Chemistry, Volume 63, Issue 11, Pages 1680–1683, https://doi.org/10.1373/clinchem.2016.268839.

Roberts, T. Kraft, C. French, D. Ji, W. Wu, A. Tangpricha, V. Fantz, C. (2014) Interpreting Laboratory Results in Transgender Patients on Hormone Therapy. The American Journal of Medicine, Volume 127, Issue 2, Pages 159-162, https://doi.org/10.1016/j.amjmed.2013.10.009. https://www.sciencedirect.com/science/article/pii/S0002934313008966

Filler, G. Ramsaroop, A. Stein, R. Grant, C. Marants, R. So, A. & McIntyre, C. (2016). Is Testosterone Detrimental to Renal Function?. Kidney international reports, 1(4), 306–310. https://doi.org/10.1016/j.ekir.2016.07.004. https://www.ncbi.nlm.nih.gov/pmc/articles/PMC5720528/

Horvath, H. (2021). 1207 PubMed citations on male/female sex differences. https://drive.google.com/file/d/1zm95pWo7zts_RArjXXRezSjPyBBqX6t6/view

Miller, W. G. (2017). Commentary. Clinical Chemistry. Volume 63, Issue 11, Page 1683. https://doi.org/10.1373/clinchem.2017.272708

Chapter 6

Transgender Medicine as Departure From First Principles

Transgender medicine is predicated on the idea that trans-identifying people are so biologically and psychologically unique that the usual approach medicine takes to treating patients doesn't apply to them.

For example, we know that biological sex in humans is binary, which is to say that there are only males and females. Males have X and Y sex chromosomes, they are typically bigger and stronger and have testicles and a penis which enables them to impregnate a female. Females, on the other hand, have only X sex chromosomes, they are typically smaller than males, and they have a vagina, cervix, uterus, ovaries and breasts, which allow them to become pregnant, birth and feed the young.

The sole purpose of biological sex is sexual reproduction. However, because there are thousands of gene expression differences between male and female humans (Weizmann Institute of Science, 2017), biological sex affects all bodily systems (Deegan & Engel, 2019; Heydari et al, 2022).

Sex is determined at conception when a mother's egg, which

carries an X chromosome, is fertilised by a father's sperm, which can carry either an X or a Y. From there on, as the embryonic cells divide and the embryo develops, the male or female specific karyotype (complete set of chromosomes) is replicated in every cell of the body. This is why biological sex in humans cannot be changed. To achieve a true sex change science would need to be capable of changing an X chromosome into a Y, or vice versa, and reversing all the sex-specific developmental, anatomical and physiological differences, which is simply not possible.

The only thing that modern medicine is capable of doing is modifying human bodies to superficially resemble the opposite sex, through the use of opposite sex hormones and cosmetic surgery. This might drastically alter the appearance of an individual but it doesn't change their biological sex in any way.

Despite this, transgender activists claim that medical interventions designed to masculinise females and feminise males constitute a true sex change. Alternatively, they assert that trans-identifying people were "born in the wrong body" and because of this, their sex exists on the spectrum between the body and their feelings about which sex they should be. These feelings are termed "gender identity" and the latest iteration of gender ideology asks us to believe that it is this feeling, rather than genetics and the resulting anatomy and physiology, that determines whether a person is male or female.

This is a pseudoscientific ideology based on wishful thinking. Yet, it has permeated all institutional policies, and even governments have now been mislead into believing that opposite sex-identifying people are "born as one sex but are the other sex. For example, a person who looks like a man on the outside, may be a woman on the inside." (Welsh Government, 2021)

Part of the reason why this ideology has been so successful is precisely because it is so outlandish. Virtually every doctor I spoke to about this laughed out loud when they were told what transactivists were claiming, and the same is true for the general population. Everyone knows what men and women are and, more importantly, that people can't become the opposite sex. The evidence of both the binary and immutable nature of biological sex is all around us and it underpins our entire society - especially healthcare. Therefore, for a long time, society as well as the medical profession were happy to go along with the "born in the wrong body" narrative, assuming it was just a metaphor that described the kind of psychological distress opposite-sex identifying people feel.

This has worked to the advantage of transactivists, who have used a variety of tactics designed to obfuscate basic scientific facts, in order to embed the myth of "sex change" into all spheres of life.

Redefining words

In large part, the new orthodoxy of make-believe sex changes was achieved by conflating sex and gender. The English language, which developed a convention of sex and gender being used interchangeably to refer to biological sex, made it possible for transactivists to equate the biological state of being a man, woman, male or female, with socially constructed stereotypes of masculinity and femininity.

This forced linguistic change was coupled with draconian institutional policies embedded by stealth, which prioritised the feelings of those who desired to be seen as the opposite sex, over and above the rights of others to state facts about biological sex.

Systematically, the word "woman" started to disappear from women's health, on account of being "offensive" and "exclusionary" of both men who identify as women and of women who identify as men. The word "sex" was replaced with "gender" and the requirement to state and record biological sex accurately was removed. This compromised the collection of sex-based data in all areas, including healthcare, crime statistics and government policy, and it allowed transactivists to play around with the concepts of male and female without being hindered by biology. Everything in this conversation has been redefined as a social construct, and the idea that you can manifest whatever you can imagine - that even what is medically impossible is in fact possible through strength of will and conviction alone - has taken hold. Meanwhile, women are still suffering health-based, and other types of discrimination, and trans-identifying people are having their bodies unethically experimented on. Society is just not supposed to use the words which would bring this into sharp relief, unless of course one doesn't mind being called a "hateful and exclusionary bigot" and risk the consequences of such an accusation.

False equivalence

Very rarely, genetic abnormalities of X, Y or other chromosomes, and other anomalous events that can occur during gamete production, at fertilisation or during foetal development, can result in Disorders of Sex Development (DSDs). These rare medical conditions are typically characterised by ambiguous genitalia, a mix of male and female sex characteristics and even a complete mismatch between external appearance (phenotype) and genetic sex (genotype).

In most cases, DSDs are diagnosed soon after birth but, sometimes, the diagnosis can be delayed.

For example, a child who is assumed to be a girl from birth can fail to start menstruating. When she is investigated she is found to have a 46 XY male karyotype, internal testes and an absence of uterus or ovaries, which would be consistent with a diagnosis of Complete Androgen Insensitivity Syndrome (CAIS). Or a child who was assumed to be a boy can present in adolescence with short stature, small testicles and gynaecomastia. When he is investigated he is found to have a 46 XX female karyotype and non-functioning testicles, which is consistent with a diagnosis of a 46 XX testicular disorder or De la Chapelle Syndrome.

In other cases, a child who is born with a DSD can be raised as the opposite sex - a practice known as "assigning sex".

Depending on a variety of factors, people with DSDs can develop an opposite sex "gender identity" and this has given rise to phrases such as "46 XY female" or "XX male syndrome" in medical literature. Any clinician reading such a paper will not be confused about the biological sex of the patient. They will simply make a mental note of genetic sex, while understanding that the way the patient perceives themselves is more in accordance with the way they look and how they are treated by society, than with their karyotype.

While medical practitioners are used to such nuance, the general public has taken the social convention of referring to DSD males with a female phenotype as "women and girls" and DSD females with a male phenotype as "men and boys" more literally. This has given rise to a misconception that biological sex is more accurately determined by external appearance and internal sense of "gender identity" than our genetic make up.

These complexities were misappropriated by transactivists to claim biological sex is a spectrum, that people are more or less male or female depending on how they look and that one's true biological sex can only be known through self-declared "gender identity".

I say "misappropriated" because karyotyping studies in gender clinics have shown that trans-identifying people have no higher incidence of DSDs than the general population (Pang et al, 2018; Çankaya et al, 2021). Therefore, the language used to describe the experiences of DSD patients is not applicable to normally sexed humans who, in the absence of a disorder of sex development, come to identify as the opposite sex.

When challenged, transactivists claim that it is impossible to truly know anyone's sex without "inspecting their genitals" or karyotyping them - thus denying the reality of human sexual dimorphism and the fact that accidental mis-sexing in day to day life is extremely uncommon - and they insist that the most ethical way forward is to abandon the notion of biological sex altogether and simply accept that people are whatever sex they say they are.

Disorder vs difference

All disorders are differences, but not all differences are disorders. Biological differences between males and females, for example, exist by design so that our species can reproduce. Therefore, these differences are not disorders. Disorders, by definition, interfere with normal function and they can make a person vulnerable, limit their opportunities and make them a target of social prejudice.

In a justified desire to remove the stigma attached to illness and disability, patients, social justice activists, and doctors alike have tried to move away from pathologising language. Instead of "disabled" we say "differently abled". Instead of "disorder" we are meant to say "variation". However, when we fail to use accurate language to describe things, other problems inevitably follow.

An overzealous denial of pathology in order to reduce

stigma, and the turning of pathology into something a person can choose to identify with, can lead to healthy people being unnecessarily medicalised, as well as medical patients being denied access to essential medical care. Or, to someone being medicalised for the wrong thing.

For example, we are already hearing about patients with DSDs struggling to access hormone supplementation because their clinicians have become so impressed by the "de-pathologising" arguments, they have come to believe DSDs are just a normal variation within the "sex spectrum" which doesn't need treating.

Likewise, transgender patients are not receiving psychotherapy for the psychological distress caused by their desire to be the opposite sex. Instead, their healthy bodies are being unnecessarily pathologised and irreversibly modified in an attempt to bring them closer to their erroneous self-perception.

I believe that societal guilt and shame about the harms and stigma inflicted on anyone who doesn't satisfy the Platonic ideal of what a male and female should look like (and how they should behave), played a big part in why gender ideology was so uncritically accepted. People with DSDs and disabilities, as well as feminine men, masculine women, and especially homosexuals, are all oppressed minorities that have historically suffered abuse and discrimination. However, while the desire to correct past wrongs and include all humans as equals in our society is understandable, the overcompensation has created more problems.

Just like pretending to "not see colour" doesn't actually reduce discrimination toward ethnic minorities, "not seeing a disorder" can serve to stifle attempts to address patients' unique needs.

Normal vs abnormal

It is normal for women to go though the menopause in middle age. During this period, it is not uncommon that they should experience symptoms caused by a drop in their sex hormone levels. These symptoms can be alleviated by prescribing oestrogen, or oestrogen and progestin, which is known as hormone replacement therapy or HRT.

Men who have a testicular disorder - for example if their testicles were removed or are not functioning properly due to a medical condition - might suffer symptoms due to lack of testosterone. This can be alleviated by testosterone therapy, which is designed to restore male-typical levels of sex hormones in order to prevent the long-term consequences of testosterone deficiency, such as osteoporosis.

In the area of transgender healthcare, all this is reversed.

Feminising hormone treatments prescribed to males who identify as females are currently being described as "HRT", even though these treatments do not replace normal levels of sex hormones in males. Instead, they induce a severe hormonal imbalance characterised by lack of testosterone and excess of oestrogen and sometimes progesterone.

Likewise, masculinising doses of testosterone when prescribed to females abnormally elevate their serum testosterone and cause a drop in $17\text{-}\beta$ oestradiol to post-menopausal levels (Loverro et al, 2016).

In effect, transgender healthcare induces endocrine abnormalities in trans-identified patients but, thanks to the misapplication of terms such as "HRT" for men on feminising doses of oestrogen, and "testicular disorder" for women on masculinising doses of testosterone, these interventions have been equated with sex-appropriate healthcare.

Interestingly, things don't tend to work out the other way around.

Try as a woman to go to a gynaecologist to ask them to remove your uterus and ovaries at, say, 28 years of age and you will not be approved for such an operation even if you are anaemic from excessive bleeding as a result of fibroids, in a lot of pain due to endometriosis or absolutely certain you don't want to have children.

Claim to be transgender, however, and your surgery will be booked with no quibble.

Special case pleading

Puberty is a time when humans acquire secondary sex characteristics which are difficult to reverse. Women who identify as men retain their female-typical body habitus and men who identify as women struggle to obscure masculine features, despite extensive cosmetic surgeries and cross-sex hormone treatments.

Therefore, in an attempt to devise medical protocols that would make trans-identified individuals visually indistinguishable from the members of the opposite sex, the target population has become ever younger.

Puberty blockers, such as GnRH agonists, were previously prescribed to children who entered puberty very prematurely. The treatment continued for the shortest time possible and, once the child reached the age at which puberty would normally occur, the treatment was discontinued so that the puberty could proceed. Even in this cohort, puberty blocker treatment is associated with depression, anxiety and seizures and is known to cause debilitating long-term side effects, such as osteopenia, osteoporosis and joint problems. (Jewett, 2017)

And yet, in the case of children with gender dysphoria, we

are supposed to believe that puberty blockers can be given for extended periods with no ill effects.

Over the last 6-7 years it has become commonplace in the field of paediatric gender reassignment to initiate puberty blockade as soon as the first signs of puberty appear. This deliberate arresting of normal development - which is advertised as a "fully reversible pause button" - continues until the child is older, when they are swapped to a cross-sex hormone regimen, with a view to having "gender confirmation surgeries" when they come of age.

In many jurisdictions cross-sex hormones can only commence when a child is 16, or older, and surgeries can only be carried out on over 18s. However, because this area of medicine is heavily influenced by the demands of transactivists, there are clinics where girls as young as 8 are being injected with masculinising doses of testosterone and having mastectomies as a part of "gender confirmation" at 13 and 14 years of age. (Transgender Trend, 2019)

There are serious concerns in the medical community over the safety of these interventions. Puberty is a natural stage that is crucial for our cognitive, sexual and bone development. It is also the time when our sexuality and identity are formed and it's a necessary stage a child goes through in order to develop into a healthy adult.

Therefore, it is medically absurd to claim it is safe to never allow a child to go through puberty. So is the assertion that flooding children's bodies with cross-sex hormones would induce the "opposite sex puberty".

Normally in medicine, a child who fails to enter puberty is investigated to find the underlying cause. Patients of all ages who exhibit opposite sex bodily changes such as breast growth and lactation in males, or hirsutism, male pattern baldness and deepening of the voice in females, are routinely investigated to ascertain the cause of their hormone imbalance. The goal of treating all these conditions is to restore normal hormone levels. In the context of medical gender reassignment, however, we are led to believe the opposite - that doctors inducing severe hormonal imbalances for the rest of the patient's life is beneficial to a patients' health.

Paediatric gender reassignment persists as a practice despite growing evidence that children who take puberty blockers and cross-sex hormones are experiencing bone thinning, negative mood changes, stunted genital growth in boys, loss of sexual drive, anorgasmia as adults, and even sterility. Females who take masculinising doses of testosterone are reported to experience uterine atrophy, and both sexes acquire an increased risk of cancer and cardiovascular disease.

Furthermore, the younger a patient is when gender reassignment treatments are started, the earlier they will experience long-term and even irreversible side effects. Unfortunately, this doesn't appear to significantly influence policies that are supposed to regulate this practice. Instead, false suicide statistics (Transgender Trend, 2016) are used to claim that puberty blockers and cross-sex hormone treatments are "life saving" in children with gender dysphoria, and parents who are reluctant to consent are asked whether they would rather have a dead son or a living daughter (Ridley, 2021).

Meanwhile, evidence in fact suggests the opposite - gender-reassigned children have more attendances for mental health problems (Hisle-Gorman et al, 2021) and, in adults, these treatments increase rather than decrease suicide risk. (Dhejne et al, 2011)

Good vs bad outcomes

One of the earliest attempts at "sex change" involved a male crossdresser called Lili Elbe, who underwent a series of experimental surgeries in the late 1920s, under the supervision of infamous sexologist Magnus Hirschfeld. The surgeries, which included amputation of the penis and testicles and insertion of an ovary into the abdominal musculature, culminated in 1931 with an implantation of a uterus and the creation of a pseudo-vaginal canal, in the hope that this would allow Elbe to realise his dream of giving birth to a child.

Despite these surgeries eventually leading to Elbe's death in September 1931, he wrote: "But that I, Lili, am vital and have a right to life I have proved by living for fourteen months. It may be said that fourteen months is not much, but they seem to me like a whole and happy human life. The price which I have paid seems to me very small. If sooner or later I should succumb physically, I am quite reconciled. I shall at least have known what it is to live."(Elbe, 1933)

Apparent patient satisfaction notwithstanding, in medicine, we would not consider this a good outcome.

However, in the area of gender reassignment, patient satisfaction - or rather an absence of evidence of dissatisfaction - remains one of the main claimed parameters of success to this day. It doesn't seem to matter that many patients have serious post-operative complications, early strokes and heart attacks, infertility, permanent sexual dysfunction and cognitive and bone problems. If they say they are happy and don't complain - or indeed if they are lost to follow-up or prevented from complaining officially due to ideological hostility toward gender reassignment regretters - it all counts toward "satisfactory outcomes".

Meanwhile, essential research is being stifled, such as in the case of psychotherapist James Caspian who had his application to research detransition (gender reassignment reversal) declined by one UK university, "because it was 'potentially politically incorrect' and would attract criticism on social media". (Weale, 2017)

The resulting lack of robust and unbiased data allows trans-activists to continue claiming that detransition, and transition regret, hardly ever happen, even while quoting studies on outcomes post gender-reassignment where loss to follow-up is unacceptably large - between 15 and 75%. (Horváth, 2018).

In any other area of medicine, loss to follow-up rates larger than 20% - or indeed smaller than this depending on the worst-case scenario - are understood to severely compromise the study's validity (Dettori, 2011). Therefore, the field of medical gender reassignment is quite unique in terms of poor quality evidence and the ongoing neglect of unbiased research being used to justify irreversible medical interventions on otherwise physically healthy people.

Body vs mind

The belief in a separation between mind and body is not new. Human cultures have long conceptualised mind and body as a duality in which the "pure and superior" mind is trapped in the "vulgar and inferior" fleshy cage of the body. This has given rise to the "mind over body" doctrine which has contributed to the idea that physical illness can be cured with positive thinking, as well as the idea that psychological distress can be cured by radical interventions on the body.

Transgender ideology posits that the psychological distress associated with gender dysphoria - such as suicidal ideation, depression, anxiety, delusions that one's sexed body is "wrong" and obsessions with achieving an opposite sex appearance - are just manifestations of a suffering mind that has been "born in the wrong body". Therefore, they ask that doctors treat this mind-distress not with psychological therapies that aim to help the mind accept the body as it is, but by modifying the body to fulfil the desires of the mind.

In reality, mind and body are inseparable. The mind - or our awareness and interpretation of internal and external stimuli - resides in, and is the function of, the body. Through the actions of nerves and neurotransmitters, this incredibly complex system receives input from all areas of the body and it exerts conscious control over much of it.

Given that mind and body are so intertwined, it is not uncommon for physical illness to present as a psychological symptom, or for psychological distress to manifest as a somatic complaint.

A brain tumour can cause hallucinations. Heart problems can present as anxiety. Endocrine imbalance as mood disorders. Conversely, depression can present as a headache. Delusion as a sensation of parasites crawling under the skin. Panic attack as a heart attack. In extreme cases, psychological distress can even cause patients to develop a fixation on doctors performing physical interventions in order to relieve their suffering.

Body Integrity Identity Disorder (BIID) and apotemnophilia, for example, are rare psychiatric disorders in which patients seek surgeons to amputate their healthy limbs in order to help them achieve a desired disability. If they can't access these interventions, these patients are known to threaten suicide and to even go as far as attempting to carry out amputations themselves. (Elliott, 2000)

In such extreme situations, it is tempting to imagine that the patient knows best and to carry out surgical mutilation in the hope this might improve the patient's mental state. Indeed a few surgeons have offered healthy limb amputation services over the years and, anecdotally, some BIID and apotemnophilia patients reported an improved quality of life. However, the benefits of these surgeries have not been proven scientifically. Elective amputations result in disability and long-term complications, they don't necessarily resolve psychological distress and can even result in further amputation desires. Therefore, irreversible bodily damage as a cure for psychological distress is considered unethical and the treatment of these conditions instead focuses on non-invasive methods such as neuropsychological rehabilitation. (Müller, 2009; Sedda & Bottini, 2014)

Like patients with BIID and apotemnophilia attempting at-home amputations, patients with gender dysphoria are known to be taking matters into their own hands and self-medicating with puberty blockers and cross sex hormones bought from illegal online pharmacies. Unlike healthy limb amputation - which is neither encouraged nor provided by the mainstream health services - medical institutions recommend that GPs should provide "bridging prescriptions" of puberty blockers and opposite sex hormones to patients who haven't yet been assessed by specialist services, under the rationale that it is less harmful if patients obtain these drugs from legitimate sources.

Furthermore, despite laws against genital mutilation, surgeons are celebrated for amputating and mutilating healthy breasts and genitals, as long as the patient has consented and the procedure is designed to be "gender affirming".

If we don't consider the amputations of healthy body parts in cases of BIID and apotemnophilia to be ethical, why then is irreversible damage to the body, in order to fulfil the desires of the mind, seen as best medical practice for gender dysphoria?

Gender dysphoria, like most psychiatric conditions, is a result of the complex interplay of environmental factors (trauma, grief, homophobic bullying) and internal factors (autism, another mental illness or even a paraphilia), and as such, it can take a long time for the patients to recover from it, and in some cases, the illness might even be treatment-resistant.

Both medicine and psychiatry are sometimes quite straightforward. The patient comes in, the doctor promptly diagnoses what's wrong and prescribes treatment, and the patient gets cured. This ideal scenario is certainly desired by both doctors and patients. However, while most patients are likely to repeatedly experience this scenario throughout their lives - or at least in their youth - a significant proportion of every doctors' practice is devoted to patients for whom there are no easy answers. Dealing with such a patient, whose symptoms are treatment-resistant, or whose diagnosis eludes us, can make doctors feel "heart-sink" about the patient's ongoing distress and the doctor's own inability to help them.

Due to a big surge in opposite sex identification among both minors and adults in recent years, doctors are seeing an ever increasing number of distressed patients who demand a quick fix for their psychological distress. Also, transgenderism and gender dysphoria have become celebrated "identities", and access to immediate affirmation and medical gender reassignment has been couched by activists in terms of "human rights".

With psychiatric services at a breaking point and waiting lists for child and adolescent mental health assessments several years long, healthcare services are under increasing pressure to develop policies and protocols which ignore the parallels with related psychiatric phenomena, and simply fulfil the demand for medical gender reassignment. As a result, the treatment approaches have focused on an informed consent model of care and clinicians have been discouraged from exploring the reasons for an opposite sex identification. This collusion between transgender activists and health services, to treat the disorder of the mind by irreversibly altering the body, has even resulted in equating exploratory psychotherapy to "conversion therapy" and some ill-advised attempts to ban it.

The truth is, despite our intimate connection with the mind, it remains one of the least well understood bodily systems. The disciplines that deal with the mind specifically - such as psychiatry and psychology - struggle to explain many phenomena that arise in the mind, and the treatment options are even more scarce, often relying on educated guesses and trial and error. Perhaps this is why so many medical scandals arise in this area. Lobotomies, insulin shock therapies and cosmetic body modifications are all failed attempts to cure psychological discomfort, and even serious psychiatric illness, with quick fix physical interventions.

The urge to help distressed patients is completely understandable. Doctors, including psychiatrists, are optimistic to a fault. They are reluctant to give a bad prognosis or to simply give up. However, just like treating a desire to be disabled by cutting off healthy limbs, treating the desire to be the opposite sex with puberty blockers or surgery, while allowing the underlying psychological issues to go unaddressed, is likely to do more harm than good.

A way forward

Medicine often involves managing patient expectations and this is where an approach that largely ignores the mind, when met with the excessive optimism of doctors, can spiral into unethical practices.

Genital surgery as a part of gender reassignment, for example, involves the removal of normal and healthy organs and the construction of poorly functioning simulacrums which are meant to replace them. This isn't always clearly communicated to the patient. I have heard surgeons who operate in this field claim that they are in fact "constructing genitals", and gender reassignment patients say their neo-genitals are the same as natural genitals.

The truth is that a surgeon would fail an exam if they claimed a surgical cavity which has to be dilated in order to prevent it from healing over is the same as an embryologically developed vagina, or that an artificially created phallus which has to be inflated through a pump and which lacks the urethra, is the same as a penis.

Doctors involved in gender reassignment are also known to claim that they are changing people's sex, even though not one of their interventions is capable of re-writing our genetic code, reversing our sexual development or redesigning bodies to perform full reproductive functions of the opposite sex. When confronted with reality, these doctors often resort to transactivist arguments, such as equating gender-reassigned men with post-menopausal women, and asking whether a woman stops being a woman if she is no longer fertile, as if that's some kind of "gotcha" that proves sex in humans can be changed. By doing this, they ignore normal human physiology, the way it naturally changes over time, and the difference between males and females, as well as between normal and abnormal.

I have no statistics on the personality profiles of doctors who promote medical gender reassignment, but I have noticed that some of them seem enamoured with their own skills, and that their need to make their patients happy sometimes overrides their commitment to do no harm.

Even the most blunt and practical doctors can find themselves downplaying the negative outcomes and avoiding saying things that might upset or disappoint their patients. Doctors, generally speaking, don't like confronting their patient's illusions (or indeed delusions) and if they aren't vigilant and self-reflective, they can find themselves colluding with the irrational belief that, if only everyone tried hard enough, all would be well. When things go wrong, all too often the patient is blamed and referred elsewhere. Difficult patients end up being shuttled between the services, and this contributes to the lack of long-term follow up and robust data on long-term outcomes. This could explain why, instead of pausing the controversial practice of gender reassignment amid concerns about lack of evidence-base, the medical establishment opted to expand it from vulnerable but competent adults, to children.

"If we could only get to them young enough, the outcomes would be better", they say to an audience that is swayed by how "passable" an androgynous teenager looks in gender non-conforming clothing. The power of advertising inherent in this cannot be ignored. However, that teen will grow up, and their biology will assert itself. When this happens not only will they no longer effortlessly "pass" as the opposite sex, they will also be saddled with the consequences of surgical mutilation and iatrogenic medical conditions.

"Not to worry! We can administer more treatments, carry out further surgeries, to make things look or work better!"

But do they stop to think about what they are doing to their patients in the long run?

I can only imagine how hard it must be for anyone to decide to live with all the consequences of medical gender reassignment. To think these patients aren't being told the whole truth about the risks, benefits and limitations of these treatments is terrifying.

Ultimately, it is not the case that trans-identifying people are so different from the rest of humanity, that the normal rules of medicine and ethics somehow don't apply to them. They are simply being failed by medical professionals who promote treatments that too often result in poor outcomes, unquestioningly affirm inner feelings and offer ever faster and earlier access to drugs and surgery. Instead, clinicians should contemplate the fact that medicine may not be able to offer a cure for gender dysphoria. Or that far from being a quick fix that requires a monthly prescription and a few cosmetic surgeries, the cure might lie in addressing societal prejudices and other economic and psychosocial factors that are driving this curious body dissociation phenomenon. The first is an approach the medical profession is already coming to regret. The latter is the alternative, yet daunting, task none of us can guarantee to achieve in our lifetimes.

Perhaps, in the future, we will find a way to cure gender dysphoria as easily as curing a bacterial sore throat. We might even achieve the impossible - devise methods to truly change biological sex. Meanwhile, as professionals who gave an oath that we would first do no harm, we must try to alleviate suffering without causing unnecessary physical and psychological damage. Patients may not be happy with us, they might not get exactly what they want in the moment and they might end up resenting us for it, but we need to fulfil our ethical obligations toward them anyway.

Bibliography

Weizmann Institute of Science. (2017, May 4). Researchers identify 6,500 genes that are expressed differently in men and women: Genes that are mostly active in one sex or the other may play a crucial role in our evolution, health. ScienceDaily. www.sciencedaily.com/releases/2017/05/170504104342.htm

Deegan, D. F. Engel, N. (2019) Sexual Dimorphism in the Age of Genomics: How, When, Where. Front. Cell Dev. Biol., 06 September 2019. https://doi.org/10.3389/fcell.2019.00186

Heydari, R. Jangravi, Z. Maleknia, S. Seresht-Ahmadi, M. Bahari, Z. Salekdeh, G. H. Meyfour, A. (2022) Y chromosome is moving out of sex determination shadow. Cell Biosci. 2022 Jan 4;12(1):4. doi: 10.1186/s13578-021-00741-y. PMID: 34983649; PMCID: PMC8724748. https://pubmed.ncbi.nlm.nih.gov/34983649/

Welsh Government. (2021). LGBTQ+ action plan. Our plan to create a better Wales for LGBTQ+ people. https://gov.wales/sites/default/files/consultations/2021-08/lgbtq%2B-action-plan-easy-read-version.pdf

Pang, K. C. Feldman, D. Oertel, R. & Telfer, M. (2018). Molecular Karyotyping in Children and Adolescents with Gender Dysphoria. Transgender health, 3(1), 147–153. https://doi.org/10.1089/trgh.2017.0051

Çankaya, T. Onur Cura, D. Özkalaycı, H. Ülgenalp, A. (2021). Chromosomal Evaluation Results for Transgender Individuals and Questioning the Necessity of Karyotyping. Erciyes Med J 2021; 43(2): 166–9. https://jag.journalagent.com/erciyesmedj/pdfs/EMJ_43_2_166_169.pdf

Loverro, G. Resta, L. Dellino, M. Edoardo, D. N. Cascarano, M. A. Loverro, M. Andrea Mastrolia, S. A. (2016) Uterine and ovarian changes during testosterone administration in young female-to-male transsexuals, Taiwanese Journal of Obstetrics and Gynecology, Volume 55, Issue 5,2016, Pages 686-691, ISSN 1028-4559, https://doi.org/10.1016/j.tjog.2016.03.004

Jewett, C. (2017). Drug used to halt puberty in children may cause lasting health problems. https://www.statnews.com/2017/02/02/lupron-puberty-children-health-problems/

Transgender Trend. (2019). Johanna Olson-Kennedy and the US Gender Affirmative Approach. https://www.transgendertrend.com/johanna-olson-kennedy-gender-affirmative-approach/

Transgender Trend. (2016). A Scientist Reviews Transgender Suicide Stats. https://www.transgendertrend.com/a-scientist-reviews-transgender-suicide-stats/

Ridley, J. (2021). Parents speak out about the 'rush' to reassign the gender of their kids. https://nypost.com/2021/06/30/inside-the-rush-to-reassign-the-genders-of-kids/

Hisle-Gorman, E. Schvey, N.A. Adirim, T.A. Rayne, A.K. Susi, A. Roberts, T.A. Klein, D.A. (2021). Mental Healthcare Utilization of Transgender Youth Before and After Affirming Treatment. J Sex Med. 2021 Aug;18(8):1444-1454. doi: 10.1016/j.jsxm.2021.05.014. Epub 2021 Jul 8. PMID: 34247956. https://pubmed.ncbi.nlm.nih.gov/34247956/

Dhejne, C. Lichtenstein, P. Boman, M. Johansson, A. L. V. Långström, N. Landén, M. (2011). Long-Term Follow-Up of Transsexual Persons Undergoing Sex Reassignment Surgery: Cohort Study in Sweden. PLoS ONE 6(2): e16885. https://doi.org/10.1371/journal.pone.0016885

Elbe, L. (1933). Man Into Woman - An Authentic Record of a Change of Sex. Copyright, 1933, By E. P. Dutton & Co., Inc. All Rights Reserved: Printed in U.S.A. page 278. http://lilielbe.org/narrative/editions/A1.html

Weale, S. (2017). University 'turned down politically incorrect transgender research'. https://www.theguardian.com/education/2017/sep/25/bath-spa-university-transgender-gender-reassignment-reversal-research

Horváth, H. (2018). The Theatre of the Body: A detransitioned epidemiologist examines suicidality, affirmation, and transgender identity. https://4thwavenow.com/2018/12/19/the-theatre-of-the-body-a-detransitioned-epidemiologist-examines-suicidality-affirmation-and-transgender-identity/

Dettori, J. R. Loss to follow-up. Evid Based Spine Care J. 2011 Feb;2(1):7-10. doi: 10.1055/s-0030-1267080. PMID: 22956930; PMCID: PMC3427970 https://www.ncbi.nlm.nih.gov/pmc/articles/PMC3427970/

Elliott, C. (2000). A New Way to Be Mad. https://www.theatlantic.com/magazine/archive/2000/12/a-new-way-to-be-mad/304671/

Müller, S. (2009). Body Integrity Identity Disorder (BIID)—Is the Amputation of Healthy Limbs Ethically Justified?, The American Journal of Bioethics, 9:1, 36-43, DOI: 10.1080/15265160802588194 https://www.tandfonline.com/doi/full/10.1080/15265160802588194

Sedda, A. & Bottini, G. (2014). Apotemnophilia, body integrity identity disorder or xenomelia? Psychiatric and neurologic etiologies face each other. Neuropsychiatric disease and treatment, 10, 1255–1265. https://doi.org/10.2147/NDT.S53385

Chapter 7

Transactivist War on Reality - What They Think Studies Show vs What Studies Actually Show

In 2018, media outlets around the world reported that "transgender brains are more like their desired gender from an early age". This claim was based on a study titled 'Brain functional connectivity patterns in children and adolescents with gender dysphoria: Sex-atypical or not?' (Nota et al, 2017).

In the past people have theorised that transgenderism (which in these studies seems to be a synonym for "gender dysphoria (GD)" or "presenting as the opposite sex") arises from sex-atypical cerebral (brain) differentiation during foetal development.

More recently, resting state functional MRI (fMRI) studies done on GD adults, claim to have found some evidence of alterations in the brain networks (also called functional connectivity or FC) that are thought to play a role in own-body perception and self-referential thinking.

Brain regions that were examined include the medial prefrontal cortex, anterior insula, temporo-parietal junction, precuneus, visual network (VN), sensorimotor networks

(SMNs), default mode network (DMN) and salience network (SN).

Virtually all these regions are thought to be involved in multiple cognitive functions, such as visual perception of complex emotional stimuli (VNs), planning and execution of motor tasks (SMNs), social cognition (DMN), and cognitive-affective processing (SN). Therefore, pinpointing complex behavioural patterns - such as opposite sex identification - on scans that examine multitasking areas of the brain, is tenuous at best.

Regardless, some researchers believe they have found functional connectivity patterns which might be "gender dysphoria specific" - or "associated with the subjective experiences of incongruence between gender identity and sex assigned at birth", as well as functional connectivity patterns that are "sex-atypical" - or "consistent with experienced gender".

Citing lack of similar research in children, Nota et al used fMRI to examine functional connectivity patterns in pre-pubertal children and adolescents with GD, and they compared these to age-matched non-GD (or "cisgender") controls. Pre-pubertal GD and non-GD cohorts were included in the study because puberty influences body and brain maturation, and as such it may also affect functional connectivity patterns.

The GD cohort consisted of 31 pre pubertal children and 40 adolescents. In this group, the researchers referred to males as "transgirls" and females as "transboys".

The non-GD (or "cisgender") cohort comprised 39 pre-pubertal and 41 adolescent girls (females) and boys (males).

Pubertal stages varied in all cohorts.

All GD adolescents (but no other children) were on the puberty blocker treatment triptorelin.

Sexual orientation of each participant was assessed by asking whether they had ever been in love with somebody and whether that person was a boy or a girl.

In the adolescent GD cohort, almost all males and all females reported being homosexual.

In the pre-pubertal GD cohort, reported sexual orientation varied, with quite a few unknowns.

On the other hand, all non-GD (or "cisgender") adolescent and pre-pubertal controls reported being heterosexual.

Following the fMRI scans and their analysis, the authors claim to have found the following:

"In adolescent transgirls a singular, GD-specific FC pattern was found within VN-I. In addition, sex-atypical FC patterns were observed in both adolescent transgirls (SMN-II and posterior DMN) and transboys (SMN- II). In contrast, in prepubertal children diagnosed with GD we did not find any FC differences among groups."

"Our findings provide evidence for the existence of both GD-specific and sex-atypical FC patterns in adolescents with GD."

Researcher bias

From the outset, this study appears to be heavily influenced by gender identity ideology. Firstly, the authors misuse the phrase "sex assigned at birth" to describe normally sexed subjects whose sex was simply observed at birth. Secondly "gender" is never clearly defined even though terms used throughout the study, such as "gender dysphoria", "gender identity", "experienced gender", "cisgender" and "transgender", all hinge on it.

In reality, if it's not used as a polite euphemism for biological sex, "gender" refers to stereotypes of masculinity and femininity. These stereotypes are changeable across time and cultures, and, rather than being innate, they are socially constructed and used to enforce the social hierarchy in which males dominate females.

I take it that when the researchers say that biological males "experience female gender" and that biological females "experience male gender", they are referring to the subjective ideas boys with GD have of what it feels like to be a girl, and the subjective ideas girls with GD have of what it feels like to be a boy. These ideas are not rooted in reality. Because biological sex can't be changed, nobody actually knows what being the opposite sex feels like. They can only imagine it, based on individual reactions to, and experiences of, the gendered world, which are varied and highly subjective.

Likewise, diagnostic criteria for "gender dysphoria" (DSM-V, 2015) are almost entirely based on observations of gender non-conformity and individual desire to socially present as the opposite sex.

This is not to say that individual experiences of gender are irrelevant and that these experiences aren't shared. The male sex class is socialised into behaviours and practices which maintain their dominant social position (masculinity), while the female sex class is socialised into behaviours and practices that maintain their subordinate social position (femininity). Masculinity and femininity are rigid and prescriptive boxes nobody fits squarely into, but everyone feels the pressure to conform with. The resulting tension between the sex classes, and between individuals and their assigned gender roles, affects human relationships and behaviours.

However, this is not what this study purports to be examining. In fact, there is no exploration of the complexities of gendered experience at all. Instead, the researchers hypothesise that the ill-defined, mostly cultural phenomenon of "gender dysphoria" - ie. individuals attempting to relieve distress associated with gendered socialisation and gender hierarchy by emulating gender stereotypes associated with the opposite sex - has a neurobiological basis.

This hypothesis, which is rooted in assumptions that behavioural differences between males and females are innate, that they can be located in our brains and that individuals who display behaviours stereotypically associated with the opposite sex have "opposite-sex brains" is likely to be junk science (Fine, et al., 2019).

Male brains have cells that contain the Y chromosome, and these brains are only found in male bodies. Female brains are made up of cells that lack the Y chromosome, and they are only found in female bodies.

Since humans are a sexually dimorphic species - males are typically larger, stronger and have more muscle mass than females - there are some anatomical and physiological differences between the sexes, which are reflected in brain size and some brain features. However, once size differences are controlled for, human brains appear to be mosaics of features. Some of these features are more commonly found in men, others in women, but they also overlap between the sexes. (Hamzelou, 2015)

Therefore, overlapping, or "sex-atypical", features are unlikely to be the sole cause of psychiatric and socio-cultural phenomena amalgamated under the term "gender dysphoria".

Confounding factors

The findings in this study are interesting, especially considering that researchers recognised important limitations, such as the questionable relevance of self-reported sexual orientation in such young subjects and the effect of puberty blockers on the results. However, I think the conclusion that "transgender brains are more like their desired gender from an early age" is fundamentally flawed. Therefore, I would like to explore the relevant unmeasured or inadequately explored variables that could have influenced the supposed cause and supposed effect.

Homosexuality

Considering that sexuality and sexual orientation only start to develop in puberty, I agree with the researchers that self-reported sexual orientation, especially of the younger subjects in this study, is of questionable value. However, longitudinal studies show that the majority of children - and especially boys - who identify as the opposite sex in childhood and adolescence grow up to be homosexual or bisexual (Singh et al, 2021). Therefore, the effect of nascent homosexuality is relevant to some GD children in this study.

Although the positive findings were interpreted as "adolescent transgirls showing FC patterns similar to their experienced gender (female)" and "adolescent transboys showing a FC pattern similar to their experienced gender (male)" all we can really say is that in this small study, puberty blocked, mostly homosexual, adolescent boys showed some functional connectivity patterns that were either unique or similar to non-puberty blocked heterosexual adolescent female controls. Likewise, puberty blocked, homosexual adolescent girls showed some functional connectivity patterns similar to non-puberty blocked heterosexual adolescent male controls.

This is significant in the light of the existing evidence that brain scans of gay men and heterosexual women (Savic & Lindström, 2008), as well as lesbian women and heterosexual men (Berglund et al, 2006), may share some similarities.

Looking at the previous research, I found another study which reported similar findings, where the authors acknowledged that "sexual orientation of the participants with GD might present a confounding factor. Berglund et al. showed that hypothalamic responsiveness to androstadienone in lesbian women was comparable to that of heterosexual men. In the literature, the majority of natal females with GD are reported to be gynephilic, which was true as well for our group of adolescent dysphoric girls. Therefore, it cannot be ruled out that the resemblance in hypothalamic activation with the control boys might be due to their shared sexual orientation rather than shared gender identity." (Burke et al, 2014)

While the framing here is incorrect - homosexual girls and heterosexual boys do not share a sexual orientation, they are simply both attracted to females - the functional connectivity similarities between these groups could be attributed to homosexuality in the GD cohort, and/or the shared attraction to a certain sex that they have in common with their heterosexual counterparts.

Mental health co-morbidities

The authors claim that a cohort of mostly homosexual, puberty blocked, GD adolescent males showed especially heightened connections in areas associated with motor control and negative emotion processing, and they "speculate that prolonged distress, such as negative self-perception and psychosocial stress due to GD may lead to alterations of FC between brain regions involved in emotional (visual) processing."

Again, the issue here is the framing of these findings as being caused by gender dysphoria, even though there are other factors that could be responsible for prolonged distress and negative self-perception.

Gay adolescents, for example, often report distress associated with homophobic bullying, and one study has found that "homophobic name calling emerged as a form of peer influence that changed early adolescent gender identity, such that adolescents in this study appear to have internalized the messages they received from peers and incorporated these messages into their personal views of their own gender identity."

Therefore, experiencing homophobic name calling predicted identifying significantly less with own-gender peers and marginally more with other-gender peers over the course of an academic year. (DeLay et al, 2018)

Furthermore, children who are diagnosed with gender dysphoria often have other mental health problems, such as body dysmorphia, eating disorders, trauma, depression, anxiety and autism. (Kaltiala-Heino et al, 2015; Holt et al, 2016)

Not only do all these conditions cause prolonged distress and negative self-perception, they could well give rise to altered functional connectivity patterns in areas of the brain that play a role in own-body perception and self-referential thinking.

In fact, psychological distress is not all that uncommon in adolescence, and certain groups - such as girls, and gender nonconforming and neurodivergent children in general - are particularly vulnerable to it.

With the "affirmation-only approach", children who are being diagnosed with "gender dysphoria" and put on puberty blockers - like the adolescent GD cohort in this study - are often not being thoroughly psychologically assessed. This has created so many problems, we are now seeing a growing number of young adults who are saying their complex mental health needs were disregarded in favour of the quick affirmation of their self-declared gender identity, and the initiation of an irreversible medical pathway that led to iatrogenic harm (Quincy Bell and Mrs A vs The Tavistock and Portman NHS Foundation Trust, 2020).

Many of these young people are now desisting from trans-identification, and historically - before paediatric gender reassignment became the norm - desistance rates were as high as 89% (see Detransition data in references at the end of essay 10). This raises even more questions regarding any proposed neurobiological basis for "gender dysphoria" and "gender identity".

For all these reasons, it is impossible to rule out mental health co-morbidities as a more plausible explanation for the altered FC patterns found in this study.

Puberty blockers

In this study, all GD adolescents were on puberty blockers (GnRH agonists). These drugs suppress the levels of sex hormones and interfere with normal physical and sexual development.

There isn't enough research to illuminate how puberty blockers given to children with "gender dysphoria" can affect cognition. However, animal studies show that GnRH agonists permanently affect cognition in sheep, especially long-term spatial memory performance. This suggests that the period during which normal puberty occurs may represent a critical period of hippocampal plasticity. Therefore, blocking or delaying normal puberty may disturb normal hippocampal formation, which could have long-lasting effects on other brain areas and various aspects of cognitive function. (Hough et al, 2017).

Research also shows that although gender dysphoria often subsides with the onset of puberty, in 98% of GD children who are given puberty blockers, it persists (Carmichael et al, 2021).

Therefore, persistent gender dysphoria, and associated distress, might have an iatrogenic, rather than neurobiological, basis.

Discussion

Research into the transgender phenomenon is both fascinating and important. Humans are curious about why males and females are treated so differently in our society, and we have grappled for centuries with trying to understand how much of this is due to nature and how much of this is due to nurture. Brain scan studies in this area are of very limited value, not only due to inherent issues with locating complex behaviour in the brain, but because the entire process is plagued by biases that are held by both researchers and the general public (O'Connor et al, 2012). This has led to unjustifiable leaps of logic and an eagerness to embrace conclusions regarding the neurobiological basis of gender dysphoria, despite existing research being of low quality (Payne, 2018).

It is perhaps not accidental that studies that aim to prove the biological basis for transgenderism focus on research that is obscure, non-specific and difficult to understand even for medical professionals. Doing so makes conclusions derived from such studies more difficult to refute, especially due to the widespread societal belief that gender stereotypes are innate. However, one doesn't need to be an expert in a specific field in order to critically appraise research and assess its validity.

Critical appraisal is a skill that has to be learned. When I was first introduced to it in medical school, I struggled because I lacked medical knowledge and clinical experience. As time went on, it got easier, until one day, ensuring that results were statistically significant, that conclusions are supported by results, that biases and confounding factors have been accounted for and that the findings are relevant to my patient population, became not only second nature but an essential skill in a profession that is vulnerable to unethical, profit-motivated research.

While there is no shame in most transactivists not having the skills required to critically appraise scientific research, their ignorance coupled with their ideological bias makes them susceptible to believing in pseudoscience. Especially if it aligns with their suppositions.

Ideological beliefs within the transgender community state that gender identity is innate, that biological sex is "fluid" and that one can be "born in the wrong body". They also believe that the only way to resolve the distress associated with being male or female in a highly unequal, gendered world is to carry out drastic body modification to help patients resemble the opposite sex. These beliefs - known as gender identity ideology - make transactivists largely impervious to any information that doesn't validate their world view. They also make them ideal foot soldiers who can be trusted to relentlessly promote false narratives and to drown out any voices that dare question their dogma.

I do not envy the researchers who are interested in exploring the neurobiological origins of gender dysphoria. They are forced to operate in a febrile and highly politicised climate, where certain conclusions are rewarded with fame and further funding, while others can jeopardise their careers. Ultimately, hope of future funding, adulation from transactivists and media exposure are not arbiters of good science. If anything, such incentives can compromise the integrity of the scientific method and I would argue that in this field, especially, meticulous attention should be paid to methodology and bias in order to avoid compounding existing problems.

Bibliography

Nota, N. M. Kreukels, B. den Heijer, M. Veltman, D. J. Cohen-Kettenis, P. T. Burke, S. M. & Bakker, J. (2017). Brain functional connectivity patterns in children and adolescents with gender dysphoria: Sex-atypical or not?. Psychoneuroendocrinology, 86, 187–195. https://pubmed.ncbi.nlm.nih.gov/28972892/

DSM-V. (2015). The DSM-5 Diagnostic Criteria for Gender Dysphoria. https://www.researchgate.net/publication/296700032_The_DSM-5_Diagnostic_Criteria_for_Gender_Dysphoria

Fine, C. Joel, D. & Rippon, G. (2019). Eight Things You Need to Know About Sex, Gender, Brains, and Behavior: A Guide for Academics, Journalists, Parents, Gender Diversity Advocates, Social Justice Warriors, Tweeters, Facebookers, and Everyone Else. S&F Online. https://sfonline.barnard.edu/neurogenderings/eight-things-you-need-to-know-about-sex-gender-brains-and-behavior-a-guide-for-academics-journalists-parents-gender-diversity-advocates-social-justice-warriors-tweeters-facebookers-and-ever/

Hamzelou, J. (2015). Scans prove there's no such thing as a 'male' or 'female' brain. New Scientist. https://www.newscientist.com/article/dn28582-scans-prove-theres-no-such-thing-as-a-male-or-female-brain/

Singh, D. Bradley, S.J. Zucker, K.J. (2021). A Follow-Up Study of Boys With Gender Identity Disorder. Front Psychiatry. 2021 Mar 29;12:632784. doi: 10.3389/fpsyt.2021.632784. PMID: 33854450; PMCID: PMC8039393. https://pubmed.ncbi.nlm.nih.gov/33854450/

Savic, I. & Lindström, P. (2008). PET and MRI show differences in cerebral asymmetry and functional connectivity between homo- and heterosexual subjects. pnas.org. https://www.pnas.org/content/105/27/9403

Berglund, H. Lindström, P. Savic, I. (2006) Brain response to putative pheromones in lesbian women. Proceedings of the National Academy of Sciences May 2006, 103 (21) 8269-8274; DOI: 10.1073/pnas.0600331103. https://www.pnas.org/content/pnas/103/21/8269.full.pdf

Burke, S. M. Cohen-Kettenis, P. T. Veltman, D. J. Klink, D. T. & Bakker, J. (2014). Hypothalamic response to the chemo-signal androstadienone in gender dysphoric children and adolescents. Frontiers in endocrinology, 5, 60. https://doi.org/10.3389/fendo.2014.00060

DeLay, D. Lynn Martin, C. Cook, R. E. & Hanish, L. D. (2018). The Influence of Peers During Adolescence: Does Homophobic Name Calling by Peers Change Gender Identity?. Journal of youth and adolescence, 47(3), 636–649. https://pubmed.ncbi.nlm.nih.gov/29032442/

Kaltiala-Heino, R. Sumia, M. Työläjärvi, M. Lindberg, N. (2015). Two years of gender identity service for minors: overrepresentation of natal girls with severe problems in adolescent development. Child Adolesc Psychiatry Ment Health. 2015 Dec;9(1):9. https://capmh.biomedcentral.com/articles/10.1186/s13034-015-0042-y

Holt, V. Skagerberg, E. Dunsford, M. (2016). Young people with features of gender dysphoria: Demographics and associated difficulties. Clin Child Psychol Psychiatry. 2016 Jan;21(1):108–18. https://pubmed.ncbi.nlm.nih.gov/25431051/

Quincy Bell and Mrs A vs The Tavistock and Portman NHS Foundation Trust. (2020). EWHC 3274 (Admin). Case No: CO/60/2020 https://www.judiciary.uk/wp-content/uploads/2020/12/Bell-v-Tavistock-Judgment.pdf

Hough, D. Bellingham, M. Haraldsen, I.R. McLaughlin, M. Robinson, J.E. Solbakk, A.K. Evans, N.P. (2017). A reduction in long-term spatial memory persists after discontinuation of peripubertal GnRH agonist treatment in sheep. Psychoneuroendocrinology. 2017 Mar;77:1-8. doi: 10.1016/j.psyneuen.2016.11.029. Epub 2016 Nov 30. PMID: 27987429; PMCID: PMC5333793. https://www.ncbi.nlm.nih.gov/pmc/articles/PMC5333793/

Carmichael, P. Butler, G. Masic, U. Cole, T. J. De Stavola, B. L. Davidson, S. Skageberg, E. M. Khadr, S. Viner, R. M. (2021). Short-term outcomes of pubertal suppression in a selected cohort of 12 to 15 year old young people with persistent gender dysphoria in the UK. https://doi.org/10.1371/journal.pone.0243894

O'Connor, C. Rees, G. & Joffe, H. (2012). Neuroscience in the Public Sphere. Neuroview, Volume 74, Issue 2, Page 220-226. https://www.cell.com/neuron/fulltext/S0896-6273(12)00330-3

Payne, D. (2018). Casualties of a Social, Psychological, and Medical Fad: The Dangers of Transgender Ideology in Medicine. Public Discourse. https://www.thepublicdiscourse.com/2018/01/20810/

Chapter 8

The Impostor Fantasy

The internet allows people to embody any identity they desire, but in virtual space only. Removed from face to face contact and other's immediate scrutiny, we can all be the little wizard behind the curtain, using magic tricks to convince others we are something we are not.

Photoshopping pictures to make models appear younger, thinner and more desirably proportioned has been affecting the self-confidence, identity and aspirations of women and girls for decades. Yet, it wasn't until these tools became available through smartphone cameras, image processing apps and social media, that people of all ages and backgrounds could create disembodied representations of their idealised selves and present them to the world.

As complex and capable as the human brain may be, it can struggle to separate reality from fiction, especially if the fiction is immersive and reinforced by life-like images and peer validation. This is why the practice of impersonating the opposite sex has been particularly successful online. Not only is such fiction impossible to dispute without the benefit of direct observation, it is easier to virtue signal theoretical acceptance when we are removed from the real-life impact trans-identification can have on the rights of others.

In face to face interactions, however, things are more complicated.

Our brains have evolved to recognise patterns and this is particularly relevant to identifying other people's biological sex. It's not only our eyes but other senses, including smell, hearing and instincts, that help us determine whether someone is male or female. This means that as well as a man may "pass" for a woman online, in real life he is invariably less successful.

Since male violence is an enduring problem in human society, various social behaviours and systems have evolved to mitigate this. Single-sex facilities and services, for example, seek to limit the access of men to women, when women are vulnerable to assault. It is particularly important to protect women, because male physical strength advantage means a woman has little chance to fight off an attack by a man. Also, women are overwhelmingly the targets of male sexual violence.

Therefore, a man cannot expect society to simply play along with his personal fiction of "being as a woman". Instead, he needs to be mindful of the boundaries of others, and if he isn't, this will lead to conflict.

Considering a widespread lack of insight into the way gender self-identification affects women, it is unsurprising that the internet is filled with angry testimonies from men, who are distressed about not being perceived and treated as if they were women in real life. Their rage is particularly directed at female characteristics they cannot possess, such as delicate features, smaller stature, small hands and feet, broad hips, higher voices and women's ability to menstruate, get pregnant and breastfeed.

Their idea of what it means to live a life in a female body is informed by the male gaze, gender stereotypes and porn. This is why their fantasy recreation of a woman hardly ever involves being paid less, doing unpaid domestic labour or being ignored. Instead they are drawn to the stereotype of beautiful bimbos whose lives are easy and filled with acceptance, slumber parties, gossiping in female toilets, colouring each other's hair and prancing around in sexy lingerie and fluffy slippers.

Meanwhile, women who don't fit feminine stereotypes are dehumanised as being "less of a woman" than trans-identifying men, and in a typically male fashion, these men talk over us, dismiss us and define us in any way that serves them.

This is one of many reasons why so many women object to men self-identifying as women. We were already struggling with misogyny, and now a group of men have stolen our name and are using their social privilege to debase us as nothing more than the figments of male imagination.

However, in this process, they are debasing themselves too.

Go down the TikTok rabbit hole and you will find lots of footage of trans-identifying men in dishevelled rooms prancing around in ill-fitting skirts and badly applied make up. Explore Reddit and you will find that many such men feel guilty about resenting women, too. The overwhelming sense of being trapped in a fantasy that has at some point spiralled into a nightmare, permeates many of these accounts.

Despite what these men might think of women like me, my heart goes out to them. So I would like to take this opportunity to offer some friendly advice, human being to human being.

Being an impostor is hard work. You have to imitate someone else, always chasing their look, their style, their experiences, and you have to work tirelessly to fool others that you are something you are not. That feeling you describe, of being uncomfortable and transgressive in your "female identity" is an internal warning sign that you are doing something wrong. That you are hurting yourself and others.

Identifying *with* someone else is empathy. Identifying *as* someone else is identity theft. You must maintain the mask at all times, because even a tiny slip is perceived as a huge inconsistency by others. When others see through the layers of your self-deception, you are overwhelmed with shame. So you end up resenting the original, because they are effortless at being themselves, forgetting that you could be yourself, too.

You could be a man who loves to wear dresses and makeup, a man who isn't macho. It would be hard to explain this to other men, but that effort is nothing compared to the effort of pretending to be a woman. You, and everyone around you, knows that you are a man. On some level you understand that no amount of pretending, demanding, crying and threatening, nor the power of state, law and medicine, can make you into a completely different human being.

When we don't like ourselves, imagining being someone else who is more successful, richer or more feminine can be very tempting. This is an escapist fantasy. We can never truly know what being in a different body would feel like. All we can do is project our pain and desires onto others and convince ourselves that the person whose life or appearance we covet, doesn't struggle with the same things we struggle with.

Doctors see this in cosmetic medicine all the time. A patient who is deeply insecure can come to hate her lips. So she pays to have fillers injected and overnight she changes her appearance. A dream come true? Not quite. When people externalise deep-seated insecurities in this way, changing the body doesn't erase the insecurity, it only makes the insecurity attach itself to something else. Eventually, displacing psychological issues erodes that person's health and sanity, because whether they have fake lips or a fake identity, they haven't addressed the underlying cause.

Self-acceptance can't be outsourced to material things or body modification. As long as we are choosing that path, we are setting ourselves up for failure. It's never about the nose, or weight, or identity. The insecurity is rooted in painful experiences, betrayal and rejection.

When I was little, I was growing up in an abusive household. Both my parents beat, berated and rejected me. I remember sitting in a bath alone, a rare moment of peace for me, wishing so hard to be prettier, thinner, more graceful. I internalised the violence of my parents, which I could neither understand nor control, and figured that if only I was less objectionable to their eyes, they would treat me better, love me more. Becoming some other girl that would not provoke their rages, was more manageable than accepting the senseless violence. I was prepared to trade my intelligence, good grades, sporting ability and health, for beauty. This led me into an eating disorder and a life of self-neglect. My body was my enemy, the reason for my suffering, and if only I could become someone else, then people would finally stop hurting me. Chances are, if you are driven to this, you have been hurt and let down too.

Whether we've been seduced into dealing with our insecurities in this way or naturally gravitate towards it, we will suffer as long as we keep pretending.

We will only know true happiness when we can look at ourselves in the mirror without judgement and embrace every part of our being - including the parts that feel heavy, distressing, and alien to us. That unconditional love toward oneself is what brings inner peace.

Chapter 9

CASE STUDY 2 - Experiment of Induced Lactation in a Trans-identifying Male

In 2018, media outlets all over the world reported on a case study where a doctor, and a nurse, at a clinic in the United States used a cocktail of drugs to enable a male patient, who identified as a woman, to breastfeed a newborn baby (Reisman & Goldstein, 2018). A UK expert commented that this was "exciting" research which could lead to more cases of "transgender women" breastfeeding (Therrien, 2018).

According to Reisman & Goldstein, the male patient (who is referred to as a "she" throughout the study) claimed that his partner - the baby's mother - was pregnant but not interested in breastfeeding, and that he was hoping to take on the role of being "the primary food source" for this infant. However, reading the paper, I could not find any evidence that the authors interviewed the mother to verify their patient's claims, or that they obtained informed consent from the mother by discussing the risks that male drug-induced galactorrhoea (nipple discharge unrelated to milk production during pregnancy and breastfeeding) could pose to the baby.

They did report that their patient had a history of "gender incongruence" but had had no gender reassignment surgeries, which means he was a fully sexed male at the time of the study. His "gender-affirming regimen" included spironolactone (a heart medication used in this case as an androgen blocker), estradiol and micronised progesterone. He was also taking occasional clonazepam and zolpidem for a panic disorder and insomnia.

At the initial appointment the patient had gynaecomastia (an abnormal enlargement of a man's breasts usually due to a hormonal imbalance or the result of hormone therapy), which was likely a side effect of the spironolactone and cross-sex hormones he was taking.

His serum testosterone level on initial examination is unclear because two markedly different values were given: 256 ng/dL in the body of text and 20.52 ng/dL in the results table 1. The authors reported no further testosterone data, which indicates that they did not measure the patient's testosterone level at any other point in the study.

In order to make sense of this glaring inconsistency, I took into account the evidence that three-quarters of trans-identified men on spironolactone and estradiol fail to reach testosterone levels within the female range (Liang 2018). I concluded that the higher figure is likely to be correct, and that this patient's testosterone was not adequately suppressed despite the authors emphasising that androgen blockade was an important part of the prescribed regimen.

While the testosterone level of 256 ng/dL might be slightly low for a man (normal male range is 265 - 923 ng/dL), it still far exceeds the normal female testosterone range of 15-70 ng/dL. In cases of Polycystic Ovarian Syndrome (PCOS) the female testosterone levels are increased, but still lower than 150 ng/dL, whereas female testosterone levels that exceed 200 ng/dL are suggestive of an ovarian or adrenal tumour (Sheehan, 2004).

There's a paucity of research into the effects of elevated testosterone on breast milk and breastfed infants. In one case report, a post-partum woman with depressive symptoms was given testosterone, both orally and vaginally (doses unknown), as well as subcutaneously via a 100 mg testosterone pellet, to improve her mood. The study concluded that "testosterone was very low in infant blood at baseline and during testosterone therapy by pellet implant. There were no adverse clinical effects in the infant after seven months of continuous testosterone therapy to the mother by subcutaneous pellet implant. Testosterone delivered by sublingual drops, vaginal cream, and pellet implant was absorbed but not measurably excreted into breast milk" (Glaser et al, 2009). However, crucial details are missing from this study - such as the age and sex of the infant, as well as the extent of breastfeeding.

Another case study concerns a trans-identified female patient (described as a "transgender man") resuming weekly testosterone injections at 13 months post partum, as a part of her "gender affirming therapy". This study showed that "milk testosterone concentrations also increased with a maximum concentration of 35.9 ng/dl when the lactating parent was on a dose of 80 mg subcutaneous testosterone cypionate weekly. The calculated milk/plasma ratio remained under 1.0 and the calculated relative infant dose remained under 1%. The infant had no observable side effects, and his serum testosterone concentrations remained undetectable throughout the study period." (Oberhelman-Eaton, et al., 2022)

This study likewise did not report the extent of the breastfeeding, and significantly, the infant in this study was male and 13 months old.

We already know that elevated testosterone in pregnant women inhibits breastfeeding, and it exposes foetuses to an hyperandrogenic environment in the womb (Barry, 2010). This can cause a variety of medical complications in girls, such as polycystic ovaries, insulin resistance and Congenital Adrenal Hyperplasia, as well as increase likelihood of gender non-conforming behaviour in childhood (Phillipson, 2013).

Considering that, currently, gender non-conformance increases the likelihood of a child being diagnosed as "transgender", that this frequently results in paediatric gender reassignment, and that the effects of elevated breast milk testosterone on newborns of both sexes are not known, there are serious ethical issues here. Including with the decision, by clinicians, to enable a man whose testosterone suppression isn't adequately demonstrated to breastfeed a potentially female infant.

This brings me to another glaring omission in this report. While the authors consistently refer to their trans-identified male patient as "she", they never state the sex of the infant involved in this experiment.

In addition to my concerns about high levels of testosterone in breast milk, this male patient is also reported to have used domperidone to stimulate galactorrhoea. Domperidone is banned in the US (FDA, 2004), and is only used off-label internationally to induce lactation in women. Domperidone is sometimes used to treat reflux but it has been discontinued for use in children under the age of 12, due to potential cardiac side-effects (MHRA, 2014). When domperidone is given off-licence to stimulate lactation, it requires ensuring that the mother and infant don't have any contraindications to this treatment (Nottinghamshire Area Prescribing Committee, 2021).

There's no evidence, here, that the authors attempted to ascertain this.

There's also no evidence that the patient stopped using clonazepam, a drug that can cause sedation in infants, or zolpidem (also known as Ambien), which could exacerbate the effects of clonazepam, prior to commencement of "breastfeeding".

When we talk about the safety of medicines in breastfeeding, we weigh the benefits of mother's milk to the health of the child, and of bonding between the mother and baby, against the risks of discontinuing the medication. If it is at all possible and medically justified, mothers who take medicines that could be passed to their babies via breast milk often decide, or are advised, not to breastfeed in order to avoid adversely affecting their baby's health.

Contrast this with a man taking unnecessary medications to induce galactorrhoea, just so he can fulfil his desire to breastfeed.

A word on a male's desire to breastfeed.

Psychosexual disorders such as autogynaephilia are present in a proportion of men who identify as women, and a breastfeeding fetish can be a feature of this condition, as this excerpt from a news article written by one such man illustrates:

"Breastfeeding is freaky. Not the sucking bit. You're reading The Stranger, so odds are you've had a titty sucked at some point in your life. No, it's because when my baby attached to my breast, there was an incredible chemical cascade that ran through my entire body like lightning. Imagine the most electric thing a partner has ever done to you, then multiply it by 10. I could feel my brain rewiring, creating pathways that would permanently connect me to my child. (And yeah, I kind of got off on it. Don't judge.)" (Fried, 2017)

It should be said that there is some historical evidence of men occasionally breastfeeding babies in situations where breast milk or other adequate nourishment was not available, such as on long sea voyages after the death of a baby's mother (Swaminathan, 2007). These men would have had medical conditions that abnormally elevated their prolactin levels and caused galactorrhea - such as pituitary tumours - and would have resorted to it in a desperate attempt to keep the baby alive, not because it was their "desire" to do so despite an availability of appropriate food sources for the infant. It is thought that this helped infants survive mainly by maintaining hydration, not because it was an adequate substitute for the breast milk of lactating women.

In the wake of this study, numerous attempts were made to equate drug-induced galactorrhoea in men with the natural breast milk a mother produces after giving birth. This ideological narrative has gone so far that we have witnessed systematic replacement of the words "breast milk" and "breastfeeding" with phrases such as "chest milk" and "chest feeding", in an attempt to normalise this practice.

However, the research on the composition of male nipple discharge is very scarce, and the research into the effects of this type of fluid on infants is non-existent.

In one case study from 1981, the researchers collected monthly nipple discharge samples for 3 months, from a 27 year old man with hyperprolactinaemia and likely pituitary adenoma. They then compared these samples to colostrum (collected during the last trimester of pregnancy and 1 day post partum) and breast milk (collected between 1-12 months post partum) from normal lactating mothers. They concluded that "the concentrations of lactose, proteins, and electrolytes in the breast secretion of this man are within the range of colostrum and milk obtained from normal lactating women" (Kulski, Hartmann & Gutteridge, 1981). Looking at the results in detail, however, the lactose level in the male patient's nipple discharge was nearly double that of colostrum (between 4.1 and 6.3

versus 2.34 +- 0.65 g/100ml) and sodium was just below the lower end of the normal range (39.0 - 14.0 versus 61.9 +- 16.0 nm).

More importantly, unlike mother's milk, male nipple discharge hasn't occurred as a consequence of growing a baby inside his body, and it is in no way tailored to an individual child - or any child for that matter.

Breast milk is the unique nourishment lactating mothers produce in order to sustain their own babies and protect them from disease in the weeks and months after birth, when the infant immune system is still not fully developed. First milk is called colostrum (birth - 4 days), which is a thick, yellowish fluid full of fat, vitamins and particularly rich in antibodies. Colostrum changes to a more calorific transitional milk (4 days – 2 weeks), which is high in fat and vitamins, and after that it becomes mature milk which is 90% water.

Maternal antibodies are first passed via the placenta to the baby during the last three months of pregnancy, and after the baby is born, he or she continues to receive antibodies through breast milk. As mother and baby share both the genetics and the environment, these antibodies are customised by the mother's body to offer an individually tailored passive immunity and protection from the pathogens the baby is most likely to encounter.

Therefore, I found it strange that Reisman & Goldstein made no attempt to analyse the composition of their male patient's drug-induced nipple discharge, considering that they talked at length about the benefits of breastfeeding on mother and baby, none of which were applicable to their male patient or indeed the infant he, allegedly, fed.

Be that as it may, as a consequence of a cocktail of drugs and a breast pump, this patient started to "lactate", eventually producing 8 oz of nipple discharge daily, two weeks prior to the birth of the baby.

Although we have no further details about the volume, the study claims that whatever fluid was produced, it was the sole source of this baby's nourishment for 6 weeks. After this time, the patient reportedly started to supplement with 4–8 oz of Similac brand formula daily.

The authors gave no indication that they observed this alleged "breastfeeding", or that they met the mother or the infant. They did state that "the child's pediatrician reported that the child's growth, feeding, and bowel habits were developmentally appropriate", but offered no corroborating evidence.

Considering that a 5 lb baby needs about 12 oz of breast milk or formula a day, and more as the baby's weight increases, it is extremely unlikely that any infant would survive for 6 weeks on 8 oz alone. Furthermore, mothers who are unable to breastfeed know only too well how important it is to use adequate amounts of baby formula. Failing to do so can result in serious harm to the baby.

I have no evidence that the baby who was allegedly subject to this experiment was harmed in any way. However, there are so many omissions, unknowns and missing data that I cannot help but ask, why was a trans-identified man held to a drastically different standard of infant care than actual mothers?

That this experiment was conducted by a Transgender Clinic, which neither had licence, nor expertise, to oversee the breastfeeding of a newborn, only adds to my concerns regarding ethics, safety and bias in this study.

It is my opinion that, rather than constituting "exciting" new research, this study is fraught with incomplete and misleading information, disingenuous analysis and undeclared conflicts of interest. That it was also reported as fact in the media, without any meaningful challenge from the mainstream medical community, makes me wonder if transgender research has lost sight of the bigger picture and has come to prioritise the emotional needs of trans-identified males over the welfare of women and children.

Bibliography

Reisman, T. & Goldstein, Z. (2018). Case Report: Induced Lactation in a Transgender Woman. Transgender health, 3(1), 24–26. https://doi.org/10.1089/trgh.2017.0044. https://www.ncbi.nlm.nih.gov/pmc/articles/PMC5779241/

Therrien, A. (2018). Transgender woman breastfeeds baby in first recorded case, study says. BBC. https://www.bbc.co.uk/news/health-43071901

Liang, J. J. Jolly, D. Chan, K. J. & Safer, J. D. (2018). Testosterone levels achieved by medically treated transgender women in a United States endocrinology clinic cohort. Endocrine practice: official journal of the American College of Endocrinology and the American Association of Clinical Endocrinologists, 24(2), 135–142. https://doi.org/10.4158/EP-2017-0116

Sheehan, M. T. (2004). Polycystic ovarian syndrome: diagnosis and management. Clin Med Res. 2004 Feb;2(1):13-27. doi: 10.3121/cmr.2.1.13. PMID: 15931331; PMCID: PMC1069067. https://www.ncbi.nlm.nih.gov/pmc/articles/PMC1069067/

Glaser, R. L. Newman, M. Parsons, M. Zava, D. Glaser-Garbrick, D. (2009). Safety of maternal testosterone therapy during breast feeding. Int J Pharm Compd. 2009 Jul-Aug;13(4):314-7. PMID: 23966521. https://pubmed.ncbi.nlm.nih.gov/23966521/

Oberhelman-Eaton, S. Chang, A. Gonzalez, C. Braith, A. Singh, R. J. Lteif, A. (2022). Initiation of Gender-Affirming Testosterone Therapy in a Lactating Transgender Man. J Hum Lact. 2022 May;38(2):339-343. doi: 10.1177/08903344211037646. Epub 2021 Sep 7. PMID: 34490813. https://pubmed.ncbi.nlm.nih.gov/34490813/

Barry, J. A. Kay, A. R. Navaratnarajah, R. Iqbal, S. Bamfo, J. E. David, A. L. Hines, M. & Hardiman, P. J. (2010). Umbilical vein testosterone in female infants born to mothers with polycystic ovary syndrome is elevated to male levels. Journal of obstetrics and gynaecology : the journal of the Institute of Obstetrics and Gynaecology, 30(5), 444–446. https://doi.org/10.3109/01443615.2010.485254

Phillipson, A. (2013). Girls exposed to high testosterone levels 'destined to be tomboys'. The Telegraph. https://www.telegraph.co.uk/news/science/science-news/10102686/Girls-exposed-to-high-testosterone-levels-destined-to-be-tomboys.html

FDA. (2004). FDA Talk Paper: FDA Warns Against Women Using Unapproved Drug, Domperidone, to Increase Milk Production | FDA. U.S. Food and Drug Administration. https://www.fda.gov/drugs/information-drug-class/fda-talk-paper-fda-warns-against-women-using-unapproved-drug-domperidone-increase-milk-production

MHRA. (2014). Domperidone: risks of cardiac side effects. GOV.UK. https://www.gov.uk/drug-safety-update/domperidone-risks-of-cardiac-side-effects

Nottinghamshire Area Prescribing Committee. (2021). Domperidone for Lactation Stimulation – Prescribing Information. https://www.nottsapc.nhs.uk/media/1729/domperidone-info-sheet.pdf

Fried, D. (2017). My First Time Breastfeeding My Daughter. The Stranger. https://www.thestranger.com/queer-issue-2017/2017/06/21/25225867/my-first-time-breastfeeding-my-daughter

Swaminathan, N. (2007). Strange but True: Males Can Lactate. Scientific American. https://www.scientificamerican.com/article/strange-but-true-males-can-lactate/

Kulski, J. Hartmann, P. Gutteridge, D. (1981). Composition of Breast Fluid of a Man with Galactorrhea and Hyperprolactinaemia*. The Journal of clinical endocrinology and metabolism. 52. 581-2. 10.1210/jcem-52-3-581. https://www.researchgate.net/publication/15737507_Composition_of_Breast_Fluid_of_a_Man_with_Galactorrhea_and_Hyperprolactinaemia

Chapter 10

It's Not "Woman" but "Transgender" That Is a Truly Elusive Term, And How This Relates to Statistics on Trans Youth Suicide

The "transgender umbrella"

Gender identity ideology posits that anyone who identifies as the opposite sex (or one of many novel genders) should automatically gain unrestricted access to whichever single-sex space they feel more comfortable in. To this end, women-only spaces have been redefined as "gender neutral" and they are now open to anyone who is included under the "transgender umbrella".

According to LGBTQ+ charity Stonewall, "trans" (which is short for transgender) is "an umbrella term to describe people whose gender is not the same as, or does not sit comfortably with, the sex they were assigned at birth. Trans people may describe themselves using one or more of a wide variety of terms, including (but not limited to) transgender, transsexual, gender-queer (GQ), gender-fluid, non-binary, gender-variant, cross-dresser, genderless, agender, nongender, third gender, bi-gender, trans man, trans woman, trans masculine, trans feminine and neutrois."

This alleged incongruence between "gender" and biological sex hinges on the concept of self-declared "gender identity", which is defined as a "person's innate sense of their own gender, whether male, female or something else (see non-binary below), which may or may not correspond to the sex assigned at birth."

Stonewall UK doesn't define "gender", it just states: "Often expressed in terms of masculinity and femininity, gender is largely culturally determined and is assumed from the sex assigned at birth." (Stonewall, no date)

What does "gender" really stand for in conversations about transgenderism?

When "gender" is not used as a polite euphemism for biological sex, it is understood to describe socially constructed sex-role stereotypes of appearance and behaviour imposed on males and females. These social roles and norms are fluid, culture dependent and they vary across time. A few hundred years ago, pink was a masculine colour, both girls and boys wore dresses in childhood and university education was accessible to men only. A lot has changed since then, but the hierarchy of "gender" has not.

Feminine gender is still imposed on all females from birth, and it is oppressive because it relegates them to an inferior position in society - relative to males. Masculine gender, on the other hand, still bestows social privilege on males from the moment they are born. However, if males are perceived as being feminine - or insufficiently masculine - it singles them out for abuse. Sexism, misogyny, rape culture, women's unpaid domestic labour, the gender pay gap, pornography, surrogacy, prostitution, domestic violence and homophobia all stem from this hierarchy.

Male/female sex-differences in physical strength and reproductive roles are at the root of the gendered hierarchy. Men use their superior strength to both coerce, abuse and exploit women, while women continue to be vulnerable due to their biological potential to bear young and all that this entails. In addition, men work together to maintain the social order in which women are not empowered to adequately defend or protect themselves, and their young, from male violence. Therefore, it is unsurprising that despite its apparent dedication to "queering", or transgressing, gender stereotypes of masculinity and femininity - which should theoretically facilitate greater gender equality - gender identity ideology replicates the gendered hierarchy by disproportionately targeting the sex-based rights of women and girls. This is reflected in the phrase "sex assigned at birth" which appears in most materials that promote transgenderism and gender self-identification.

Sex in humans is not "assigned at birth". As I discuss in other essays, this is a misappropriation of the medical terminology which is only applicable to some people with medical conditions that affect sex development. In everyone else - including people who identify as "trans" - sex is determined at conception and simply observed and recorded at birth.

However, by claiming that sex is "assigned" rather than observed, gender identity ideology lays a foundation for its claim that some normally-sexed people who declare an opposite-sex "gender identity" had their sex mis-identified or "wrongly assigned" at birth. This sleight of hand serves the purpose of asserting the primacy of "gender identity" over biological sex. Once this is achieved, our sexed bodies become irrelevant. Only how we feel inside matters, for all purposes, and without exception.

Gender self-identification

There are two types of identities: how we are identified by others and how we self-identify.

The first type of identity is usually objective and officially recorded. Our place and year of birth identify our nationality and our age. Our primary and secondary sex characteristics identify us as either male or female. The colour of our skin and our professional qualifications identify us as belonging to certain demographics. Official documents can be tampered with, of course, but by and large they show how others objectively perceive us.

The second type of identity is subjective. Film-buff, gardener, knitter, dog vs cat lover, are all the ways we can identify ourselves according to what is significant and important to us. These identities do not have to be recognised as factual by others. I might consider myself an expert gardener, but the Royal Horticultural Society is under no obligation to accept this, unless it is accompanied by a horticulture degree and references that confirm my experience in the field.

Despite these clear and enduring social conventions, gender identity ideology has succeeded in elevating one form of subjective identification - self-identified gender - above the objective reality of biological sex. This has given rise to a transgender rights movement, whose aims can be summarised in the following, often repeated, conversation between feminists and trans activists:

transactivist: People should be accepted and allowed to be who they are, without fear of discrimination.

feminist: Agree.

transactivist: Nobody should be forced to identify with the gender that's been imposed on them since birth.

feminist: Strongly agree! Gender boxes are unrealistic, oppressive and nobody fits into them perfectly.

transactivist: Half of all transgender people have attempted suicide. Therefore we must issue personal documents to reflect how trans people self-identify, and remove all medical and legal obstacles to accessing gender-reassignment treatments, such as puberty blockers, cross-sex hormones and various degrees of reconstructive surgery (Edinburgh ATH, 2017);

feminist: Wait, what?

transactivist: Trans people's gender identity is evidence that they were born in the wrong body.

feminist: What are you on about, mate?

transactivist: Trans women are women, their penises are female, and they are discriminated against just like all other women, so they must be given full inclusion into female-only spaces and all the initiatives designed to protect women.

feminist: Transwomen are men. Sex is determined at conception and it can't be changed.

transactivist: You are a transphobic TERF! Trans people's existence is not up for debate! Check your cis privilege while we call your employer to demand they fire you from your job.

In this climate of "no debate", not one aspect of gender identity orthodoxy can be questioned without being accused by transactivists of "denying trans people's existence" and "causing trans people to kill themselves". This hyperbolic rhetoric usually culminates in anyone who opposes replacing biological sex with gender self-identification being called a Nazi, and their adherence to science and biology as being akin to "genocide". The outcome is that dissenting voices are shut down, while gender ideology's newfangled and self-serving definitions of "woman", "sex", "gender", "hate", "rights" and "violence" are forced on the rest of society.

Forced teaming

Ever since the lesbian, gay and bisexual rights movement was expanded to include "gender identity", in addition to sexual orientation, the following have all been included under the "transgender umbrella":

- gender dysphoric men, women and children, who may or may not be homosexual or survivors of sexual trauma
- heterosexual men who are aroused by the thought of being women
- male cross-dressers
- people who believe they were "born in the wrong body"
- gender non-conforming children and adults
- children and adults who are struggling with sex or gender ambivalence in the context of mental illness
- mediocre male athletes who identify as female in order to enter female sporting competitions
- men who identify as women so they qualify for positions on all-women shortlists
- men who identify as women so they gain access to vulnerable women and girls for the purpose of voyeurism, exhibitionism or sexual violence
- male sex offenders who identify as women in order to get transferred to women's prisons

It seems odd that such an abstract, heterogenous and uniquely human concept as "transgender" should be politically and ideologically teamed up with homosexuality and bisexuality, which are minority sexual orientations found in many different animal species.

Be that as it may, since T was added to the LGB, the focus of this movement has shifted from sexual orientation to gender identity, and the acronym has grown exponentially. It currently stands at LGBTQQICAPF2K+, and hitherto unknown "genders" keep being added to it all the time. These novel "genders" are accompanied by special pronouns, which are neither sex-based nor actual words in the English language (such as xe/xem, zie/zim or sie/hir).

One might be forgiven for asking how these new genders are any different from individual personalities, interests or preferences? The answer is - they are not. However, viewed through the lens of gender identity ideology, these normal and varied human inclinations are being converted into fashionable labels, which come with their own flags, days (or months) of awareness and demands for more activism and resources.

What's more, it has become a taboo - and even a hate crime - to question the validity of these identities. Today, even questioning someone's self-identified gender can get you reported to the police, or to your employer, and it can attract prolific abuse both on social media and in real life.

However, because the "transgender umbrella" incorporates such disparate reasons for gender self-identification, questioning who is really "trans", who isn't, and what "being trans" means in material reality is not only important, it is essential. Especially if we are to assess the needs of this group as well as its impact on the rights of others.

Definitions and category errors

To define anything, we must be able to objectively determine what is 'It' that we are defining, and what is 'not-It'. Including not-It in the sample of It is a category error which results in the definition of It becoming meaningless.

This is what happened when transgender activists changed the definition of "woman" to include men. In order to mask the category error, the definition of the word "woman" had to be changed from "adult human female" to "anyone who has female gender identity". If that gender identity is different from "sex assigned at birth", the woman is "trans". If it is the same, she is "cis".

For this to work, all women would have to share an "internal, personal sense of being female". But what does this mean, in reality? A woman's understanding of her being female is based on living in a female body, experiencing its unique functions and negotiating relationships in a society where females generally have fewer opportunities and much higher risk of exploitation and sexual violence than males. How can a man know what being a female feels like, when he is not female? The answer is - he can't. He can only have an idea based on the way he perceives the opposite sex, and since every man has his own ideas, this makes the definition of "woman" elusive. What's more, given that men have traditionally viewed women as weak, submissive and empty-headed sex objects who wear dresses, make up and have long hair, men who claim to be women often emulate these feminine gender stereotypes in order to substantiate their claim to womanhood.

Members of the female sex have long considered feminine gender stereotypes to be restrictive and oppressive, and we have fought to be liberated from the constraints of compulsory femininity. Men who identify as women, however, see this struggle as a privilege only "cis women" have, because real women are recognised as women even if they don't perform femininity.

Pushing this dishonest appropriation to its logical conclusion, the gender identity movement likens itself to the Civil Rights Movement, which would only make sense if the enduring struggle for racial equality was all about white people in blackface claiming not only that they are "trans Black", but that Black people enjoy "cis Black" privilege because they don't have to perform blackface.

Category errors that redefine the members of a privileged class as members of an oppressed class are particularly pernicious because they replicate the existing social hierarchies. Men who claim to be women, for example, still exploit, abuse and subjugate women, only they do this from within the women's movement, dismantling women's right to single sex spaces and silencing discussions about uniquely female experiences. This male oppression of women has been rebranded as "feminist politics" and "arguments among women", because "trans women are women - just like tall women or Black women".

When they are asked to define "trans woman" without resorting to feminine gender stereotypes or saying "I am what I am because I say am", men who claim to be women retort that "their existence is not up for debate", and that anyone who questions whether they belong in a category "woman" is "transphobic". This is no different to priests asserting that God exists, without offering any proof other than their inner feeling and conviction, and labelling anyone who questions them as a heretic. Just like the most ardent of priests, transactivists are not only asking us to believe them, they are asking us to believe *in them* as agents of truth, who are in possession of knowledge that eludes the rest of us.

The agents of gender identity ideology have nearly destroyed the sex-based protections for women and girls, which are needed to mitigate the effects of male violence. They have also seriously stifled ethical and scientific inquiry into medical gender reassignment, which involves medications and procedures that can cause sterility, increased morbidity and mortality. This makes gender identity ideology far from an innocent phenomenon.

Medicalising gender dysphoria

Historically, there were two groups that were subjected to medical gender reassignment.

The first group were adults (predominantly men) who felt that their "gender identity" was opposite to their biological sex. Sometimes, these men had a history of gender non-conforming behaviours in childhood, however this was never diagnostic because gender non-conformity is a lot more common than transsexualism.

The second group were children who were born with atypical sex characteristics. These children were medically and surgically "reassigned" to the opposite sex - usually in infancy - and subjected to psychological interventions designed to manipulate them into developing an "opposite sex gender identity". These experiments were very harmful and unethical, and they have been widely condemned by both the public and the medical profession.

It is my belief that drawing children into the adult phenomenon of "transgenderism" has served to validate the practice of gender reassignment in adults as a valid and curative medical procedure, and to whitewash the medical scandal of paediatric sex reassignment procedures.

Asserting that children can know their "true gender identity" to be opposite to their biological sex has lent credence to the idea that opposite sex identification is innate. Conversely, the fact that some adults have sought to be medically and surgically "reassigned" to the opposite sex has been used to suggest that children claiming an opposite sex "identity" is not just a phase.

This rationale has led to medical gender reassignment being made available to anyone who says they are "transgender".

If only this approach to curing feelings worked – by improving overall quality of life, for example – we could perhaps debate whether the benefits of these procedures outweigh the risks. Unfortunately, the evidence-base for these treatments is lacking.

The biggest long-term follow up study that examined outcomes in Sweden, found substantially higher rates of suicide attempts, psychiatric hospitalisations, overall mortality and death from cardiovascular disease and suicide in sex-reassigned transsexual individuals compared to a healthy control population (Dhejne, et al., 2011).

There are no equally comprehensible and long-term studies on children. However, there are many uncertainties and even evidence of harms associated with the administration of puberty blockers and cross-sex hormones for gender dysphoria (NICE, 2021 a; NICE, 2021 b).

As for the rationale for these treatments, which claim to improve mental health outcomes, it has been documented that following "gender-affirming" medical interventions, gender dysphoric adolescents experienced *increased* need for mental healthcare for adjustment, anxiety, mood, personality, psychotic disorders, and suicidal ideation/attempted suicide (Hisle-Gorman, 2021).

These findings are very inconvenient for the proponents of transgenderism. In order to mitigate this, transactivists have resorted to claiming that "half of young trans people have attempted suicide" and that paediatric gender reassignment was a "life saving treatment" for gender dysphoria.

It turns out, this emotional blackmail tactic has been so effective that, despite the lack of evidence base, a huge number of increasingly younger children are being subjected to unnecessary medical and surgical interventions designed to make them look like the opposite sex, while gender self-identification itself has become sacrosanct in our society.

False suicide statistics

The statistic that claims "half of all young trans people have attempted suicide" can be traced to a 2011 PACE survey which set out to look at the ways mental health services could be improved for LGBT+ people. It focused primarily on suicidal ideation, attempted suicide and self-harm among young LGBT+ people, heavy drinking among lesbian and bisexual women, and body image issues among gay and bisexual men. The survey recruited 2078 people.

When assessing suicidal ideation, the study looked at respondents under the age of 26, which reduced the sample size to 485 people, 27 of whom identified as transgender.

When the results were analysed, 15 out of 27 trans-identifying respondents said that they had had suicidal ideation. (Transgender Trend, 2016)

Since the early 2000s, the National Health Service has implemented the mandatory reporting of "serious incidents". Any death by suspected suicide in a patient that is either under the care of Tavistock Gender Identity Service (GIDS) or waiting to be seen, must be reported to the Tavistock's Board of Directors. The analysis of this data shows that between 2007 and 2020, four GIDS patients died by suspected suicide: two on the waiting list, in 2016 and 2017; and two after having been seen, in 2017 and 2020. (Biggs, 2022)

One of these is a well-publicised and tragic case of an 18 year old trans-identifying female committing suicide following the prescription of cross-sex hormones by an illegal online clinic (Savva, 2019).

Consequently, Tavistock GIDS has advised parents that most children and young people seen by GIDS neither self-harm nor attempt suicide. Although GIDS patients have higher rates of self-harm than all teenagers, this rate is similar to that seen in local Child and Adolescent Mental Health Services (GIDS, no date).

Despite this, the myth of high rates of suicide in gender dysphoric youth persists, and this is still being used to drive policies and legislation in this area.

Notes on suicide

Most studies that explore the issue of trans youth suicide, focus on suicidal ideation and attempts.

However, not all suicide attempts are serious attempts to end one's life. Often, they are cries for help, and in some cases, they might even be an abuse or manipulation tactic. How we categorise and respond to them, therefore, depends on context.

This is not to say that we shouldn't act from a place of compassion, or that we should dismiss anyone who makes a suicide attempt or who voices suicidal ideation. It is just a reminder that if we're analysing risk to population groups, such as trans-identifying youth for example, we need to have good studies and a thorough understanding of what the figures mean, rather than take them at face value, or even worse, misrepresent them to suit a certain agenda.

Reports of suicide attempts can be corroborated, but suicidal ideation, which usually relies on self-reporting, is much more difficult to assess especially if we rely on self-reports from surveys rather than conducting individual psychiatric assessments. Surveys can also be skewed by asking leading questions, or by targeting specific populations who are more likely to self-report a certain symptom. This selection bias can be used to generate desired results, and to justify reverse-applying these results to a much larger population without any evidence that the two populations are comparable. To compare this to a physical symptom, it's like determining the incidence of tuberculosis in patients who are hospitalised for persistent cough, and then using those results to claim that the incidence of tuberculosis in anyone who has ever coughed would be the same or similar.

Suicidal ideation is a common symptom, less so when it's persistent. Suicide attempts are rare, and even when they occur most are not necessarily accompanied by a genuine desire to die. Serious suicide attempts which aim to end one's life are even rarer, they are almost always diagnostic of mental illness and over 90% of persons who commit suicide have diagnosable psychiatric illnesses at the time of death, usually depression, alcohol abuse, or both. (Hirschfeld et al, 1997).

Mental illness, and especially mood and anxiety disorders, are present either concurrently or at some time during their lifetime, in almost 70% of individuals with Gender Identity Disorder (Heylens et al, 2014).

This brings me to another way in which suicidality in trans youth can be misinterpreted – by implying that correlation means causation.

In psychiatry, there exists a hierarchy of diagnoses with

Mood Disorders at the top of the hierarchy, followed by Psychotic Disorders, Anxiety Disorders, Personality Disorders and Other (such as ADHD, Eating Disorders, Dissociative Disorders, Gender Dysphoria etc).

This hierarchy means that mood disorders, in addition to their own unique symptoms, can produce almost any other psychiatric symptom, and the same is true for every other diagnosis in relation to those that sit below it in the hierarchy.

Therefore we shouldn't attribute suicidal ideation to Gender Dysphoria without first excluding diagnoses such as Clinical Depression, Bipolar Disorder or Generalised Anxiety Disorder. This is especially important in the light of frequent mental health co-morbidities which are found in trans-identifying youth.

I'd also like to mention the psychiatric symptom of "ambivalence" (commonly observed in psychotic disorders), which is particularly distressing when it involves one's own body, sex, gender or sexuality. This ambivalence is not just wondering whether one might be attracted to the opposite sex; it is a symptom of disordered thinking which characterises severe mental illness.

Therefore, symptoms which - when viewed in isolation - might justify someone's inclusion under the transgender umbrella, are usually symptoms of a mental illness higher up in the diagnostic hierarchy, if evaluated from a broader mental health perspective. As a lot of mental illnesses tend to develop in youth, and are often accompanied by suicidal ideation and even suicide attempts, this clearly highlights further pitfalls of trying to attribute suicidality to "being trans".

When a clinician is mandated by law or policy to simply affirm a professed gender identity without exploring their patient's history and all possible reasons for opposite sex identification, he or she risks misdiagnosing a serious mental illness and fast-tracking a vulnerable, mentally ill patient down the path of irreversible body modifications which will negatively impact their lives in the long-term.

In the book titled *Gender, Lies and Suicide: A Whistleblower Speaks Out* - which is well worth a read - a male detransitioner, Walter Heyer, describes the negative impact a misdiagnosis of his complex mental health problems has had on his life. Those problems, which were rooted in childhood trauma, were not properly addressed.

Although ideologically captured academic and medical institutions are making proper research into the phenomenon of detransition all but impossible, a survey of female detransitioners (Stella, 2016) as well as the High Court decision in the case of Bell vs Tavistock (R (on the application of) Quincy Bell and A v Tavistock and Portman NHS Trust and others, 2020) demonstrate that harm is still being done to patients under the "affirmation-only" approach to gender confusion.

During my medical career, I've looked after several trans-identifying male patients who were admitted to the psychiatric ward on 1:1 suicide watch, due to repeated and relentless suicide attempts following "gender affirming surgery" ie. castration, penectomy and neo-vagina creation. Most of them had a history of suicidal ideation and suicide attempts, which their psychiatrists and surgeons believed could only be relieved by drastic body modification.

What has stayed with me after all these years is that they were some of the most distressed patients I have ever seen. They were not only distressed because they realised surgery hadn't cured their troubled feelings, but because they had to live with their bodies being irreversibly mutilated. It goes without saying that severe psychological distress isn't conducive to the kind of self-care most gender reassignment procedures require post-operatively. This can lead to an increased rate of complications that further impact on the patient's life in an iatrogenic (doctor-caused) vicious cycle that could've been avoided.

These patients, and many others who suffer worsening physical and mental health following gender reassignment, are currently swept under the rug while the full extent of "transition regret" is not known due to the way transactivists have stifled research under the guise of "political incorrectness" (Weale, 2017).

Erasure of gender non-conformity

Currently in the UK, there are attempts to legally ban any psychotherapeutic exploration of why individual children are distressed about their sexed bodies and gendered expectations. Quite cynically, transactivists claim that such exploration constitutes "trans conversion therapy", all the while ignoring the long-standing evidence of huge rates of desistance in children who are not medicalised. As well as the fact so many of these children grow up to be same-sex attracted (Detransition data, 1978 - 2021).

When a gender non-conforming child, who would likely grow up to be gay or a lesbian, is medically reassigned to a person who resembles the opposite sex, their innate same-sex attraction is medically "converted" into heterosexuality. This is de facto gay conversion therapy.

Therefore, I must ask: do homophobia and gay erasure - in addition to female erasure and misogyny - underpin the gender identity movement?

In this essay, I set out to illustrate why it is unacceptable for transactivists to redefine the word "woman" using vague and subjective definitions such as "trans" and "gender identity", and to use false suicide statistics in order to emotionally blackmail society into abandoning an ethical approach to gender-confused children and adults. I argued that clinicians should not be facilitating gender reassignment treatments for patients who have suicidal ideation, a history of suicide attempts and/or serious mental illness. This is not only because medical gender reassignment can make psychiatric symptoms worse but because doctors have a responsibility to protect vulnerable patients - who might be lacking insight into their illness and therefore lack capacity to consent - from making decisions that cause irreversible harm to their otherwise healthy bodies.

While there are many factors contributing to gender identity ideology's apparent fixation on dissociating the word "woman" from female biology, one possible explanation is that women, or more precisely feminists, have been the most vocal critics of patriarchal power structures, including cosmetic body modification, the gender hierarchy and the initiatives that force gender non-conforming people into rigid, gender boxes.

Instead of working to dismantle systemic injustice, and with it the gender boxes themselves, or analysing how gender stereotypes harm women and all gender non-conforming people, gender identity ideology has focused on obliterating women's rights by redefining the sex category "woman" to include biological males. A further erasure of gender non-conformity by constructing endless new and unique gender categories that individuals can conform to - whilst promoting medical interventions that either modify secondary sex characteristics to resemble those of the opposite sex or erase them altogether - is counterproductive, too. The rapid rate at which adherence to these beliefs is removing sex-based rights, and making gender non-conforming people into life-long medical patients, should give us all pause.

Bibliography

Stonewall. List of LGBTQ+ terms. https://www.stonewall.org.uk/help-advice/faqs-and-glossary/list-lgbtq-terms

Edinburgh ATH. (2017) Trans Health Manifesto. https://edinburghath.tumblr.com/post/163521055802/trans-health-manifesto

Dhejne, C. Lichtenstein, P. Boman, M. Johansson, A. L. V. Långström, N. Landén, M. (2011). Long-Term Follow-Up of Transsexual Persons Undergoing Sex Reassignment Surgery: Cohort Study in Sweden. PLoS ONE 6(2): e16885. https://doi.org/10.1371/journal.pone.0016885

NICE. (2021) a. Evidence review: Gonadotrophin releasing hormone analogues for children and adolescents with gender dysphoria. National Institute for Health and Care Excellence. https://drive.google.com/file/d/1jZ68aVpVkIlypnxIow36QYCNJtvT7tgp/view

NICE. (2021) b. Evidence review: Gender-affirming hormones for children and adolescents with gender dysphoria. National Institute for Health and Care Excellence. https://drive.google.com/file/d/1dp-H1A_eBwcGY9yuHdfPi77Wr5XlDNg1/view

Hisle-Gorman, E. Schvey, N. A. Adirim, T.A. Rayne, A. K. Susi, A. Roberts, T. A. & Klein, D. A. (2021). Mental Healthcare Utilization of Transgender Youth Before and After Affirming Treatment. The journal of sexual medicine, 18(8), 1444–1454. https://doi.org/10.1016/j.jsxm.2021.05.014

Transgender Trend. (2016) A Scientist Reviews Transgender Suicide Stats. https://www.transgendertrend.com/a-scientist-reviews-transgender-suicide-stats/

Biggs, M. (2022). Suicide by Clinic-Referred Transgender Adolescents in the United Kingdom. Arch Sex Behav. https://doi.org/10.1007/s10508-022-02287-7

Savva, A. (2019). Mum's fury after transgender suicide teen sold hormones from illegal online clinic. Cambridgeshire Live. https://www.cambridge-news.co.uk/news/cambridge-news/transgender-treatment-nhs-webberley-jayden-16504026

GIDS. (no date) Parent advice - I'm worried that my child might hurt themselves. https://gids.nhs.uk/parents-and-carers

Hirschfeld, R.M. & Russell, J.M. (1997). Assessment and treatment of suicidal patients. The New England journal of medicine, 337(13), 910–915. https://doi.org/10.1056/NEJM199709253371307

Heylens, G. Elaut, E. Kreukels, B. P. Paap, M. C. Cerwenka, S. Richter-Appelt, H. Cohen-Kettenis, P. T. Haraldsen, I. R. De Cuypere, G. (2014). Psychiatric characteristics in transsexual individuals: multicentre study in four European countries. Br J Psychiatry. 2014 Feb;204(2):151-6. doi: 10.1192/bjp.bp.112.121954. https://pubmed.ncbi.nlm.nih.gov/23869030/

Stella, C. (2016). Female detransition and reidentification: Survey results and interpretation. https://guideonragingstars.tumblr.com/post/149877706175/female-detransition-and-reidentification-survey

R (on the application of) Quincy Bell and A v Tavistock and Portman NHS Trust and others. 2020. EWHC 3274(Admin)'. www.judiciary.uk/wp-content/uploads/2020/12/Bell-v-Tavistock-Clinic-and-ors-Summary.pdf

Weale, S. (2017)University 'turned down politically incorrect transgender research'. The Guardian. https://www.theguardian.com/education/2017/sep/25/bath-spa-university-transgender-gender-reassignment-reversal-research

Detransition data:

Singh, D. Bradley, S. & Zucker, K. (2021). A Follow-Up Study of Boys With Gender Identity Disorder. frontiersin.org. https://www.frontiersin.org/articles/10.3389/fpsyt.2021.632784/full

Steensma, T. D, McGuire, J. K. Kreukels, B. P. Beekman, A. J. & Cohen-Kettenis, P.T. (2013). Factors associated with desistence and persistence of childhood gender dysphoria: a quantitative follow-up study. Journal of the American Academy of Child and Adolescent Psychiatry, 52(6), 582–590. https://doi.org/10.1016/j.jaac.2013.03.016

Singh, D. (2012). A follow-up study of boys with gender identity disorder. Unpublished doctoral dissertation, University of Toronto. https://www.frontiersin.org/articles/10.3389/fpsyt.2021.632784/full

Drummond, K.D. Bradley, S.J. Peterson-Badali, M. & Zucker, K.J. (2008). A follow-up study of girls with gender identity disorder. Developmental psychology, 44(1), 34–45. https://doi.org/10.1037/0012-1649.44.1.34

Wallien, M. S., & Cohen-Kettenis, P. T. (2008). Psychosexual outcome of gender-dysphoric children. Journal of the American Academy of Child and Adolescent Psychiatry, 47(12), 1413–1423. https://doi.org/10.1097/CHI.0b013e31818956b9

Kosky, R. J. (1987). Gender-disordered children: does inpatient treatment help?. The Medical journal of Australia, 146(11), 565–569. https://doi.org/10.5694/j.1326-5377.1987.tb120415.x

Davenport, C.W. (1986). A follow-up study of 10 feminine boys. Archives of sexual behavior, 15(6), 511–517. https://doi.org/10.1007/BF01542316

Zuger, B. (1984). Early effeminate behavior in boys. Outcome and significance for homosexuality. The Journal of nervous and mental disease, 172(2), 90–97. https://doi.org/10.1097/00005053-198402000-00005

Money, J. & Russo, A. J, (1979). Homosexual outcome of discordant gender identity/role: Longitudinal follow-up. Journal of Pediatric Psychology, 4, 29–41. https://doi.org/10.1093/jpepsy/4.1.29

Zuger, B. (1978). Effeminate behavior present in boys from childhood: ten additional years of follow-up. Comprehensive psychiatry, 19(4), 363–369. https://doi.org/10.1016/0010-440x(78)90019-6

Chapter 11

Why I Decided to Stop Using the Term "Trans Woman"

Violence against women and persecution of feminists

Ever since the Gender Recognition Act was passed in 2004, UK institutions have gradually moved away from requiring people to have Gender Recognition Certificates (GRCs) and towards allowing anyone to change the sex markers on their documents based on self-identification alone. This was achieved through the deliberate misinterpretation of the Equality Act 2010, whereby LGBT+ lobby groups persuaded institutions that it was "illegal" to ask for evidence of a GRC or to question the validity of gender self-identification.

One of the more serious outcomes of this new practice is the widespread mis-sexing of male criminals in the media, as well as crime statistics and court proceedings.

This has largely flown under the radar. While some media outlets have revelled in the apparently huge increase in the number of "women" committing sex offences, feminists who tried to bring attention to the fact that male perpetrators were allowed to self-identify as "women" were vilified as "bigots" and deplatformed. For several years, no major media outlet would publish articles where the impact of self-identification on women's safety and rights was discussed.

However, in 2017, the awareness of this abhorrent practice finally became mainstream when a young man, who self-identified as a woman, violently assaulted Maria MacLachlan, a 61 year old feminist, during an event at Speakers Corner.

Following the assault, transactivists publicly supported the assailant, and showed no compassion for the victim, while the judge compelled Maria to refer to her male attacker as "she" throughout the court proceedings. During her testimony, Maria understandably found it difficult to always remember to use her attacker's "preferred pronouns". For this, she was rebuked by the judge who said she had shown "bad grace" and although he convicted the attacker, he denied Maria compensation for sustained injuries (Moss, 2018).

Ever since then (and for sometime before it) the escalating powers of patriarchy that are embodied in the gender identity movement, have weakened women's resistance by dividing us into two categories:

1. The "trans-exclusionary" women who reject the notion that some men are women too. According to transactivists, these women deserve to be abused, threatened, assaulted, deplatformed and fired from their jobs, and they do not deserve anyone's compassion because they are "no better than Nazis".

Transactivists commonly refer to this group as "TERFS" which stands for "trans-exclusionary radical feminist". This is a misnomer because radical feminists have asserted from the very beginning that women's rights include women who identify as men ("trans men"), and have never asked for these women to be excluded in any way. What radical feminists have insisted upon is that men who identify as women ("trans women") are not women, and because of this they can be lawfully excluded from women's single-sex spaces. Therefore, the acronym "TERF" is a misogynistic dogwhistle which has been designed to punish women for refusing to accept the redefinition of the word "woman" to include men. This misogyny has been obscured to sound like a cry for "trans rights".

2. The "kind" women, who are willing to place the needs and desires of trans-identifying men above the safety of women and children. Transactivists expect these women to announce their alliance to "trans women" at every opportunity and punish them for showing any support for "TERFs", regardless of the circumstances.

Feminists commonly refer to this group as "handmaidens". This term was borrowed from the Margaret Atwood novel 'A Handmaid's Tale', which describes an extreme, misogynistic dystopia where some women are given the power to police other women on behalf of the violent patriarchy.

Most visible handmaidens today are highly paid women in politics, media, academia and the entertainment industry. These women can be seen frequently parroting gender identity ideology on social media, on behalf of their organisations, and even within their political parties. They too call other women "TERFs", claim that babies are born without a sex until one is "assigned" to them, that it is "hateful" to say the cervix is a female organ, that "transwomen are women just like Black or disabled women" and that they don't mind sharing intimate spaces with men. Handmaidens are typically not saying this while sitting in a rape crisis shelter or a women's prison but from the comfort of their middle class homes and well-paid jobs.

Meanwhile the women who are willing to stand up for

women's rights are virtually absent from positions of power, and if they happen to be in the public eye - like Joanna Cherry KC, Rosie Duffield MP, JK Rowling and Professor Jo Phoenix - they are persecuted, harassed, threatened or removed from their positions.

Owing to the tireless efforts of the grassroots feminist movement, the situation is less grim in 2022 than it was in 2017.

Thanks to the Maya Forstater judgement that ruled it was unlawful to discriminate against an employee for holding gender critical views - which is to say, knowing and being willing to publicly state that sex is binary and immutable and that men are not women - transactivists can no longer conspire to have women fired for defending their sex-based rights.

However, women still risk being attacked, in person and on social media, unless they prioritise transactivist demands while helping to police the rest of us. When pockets of resistance to gender identity ideology form in companies and institutions, the women who resist are targeted disproportionately, by men as well as other women, which leaves them feeling betrayed, vulnerable and alone.

This horrific backlash against women's rights has created a hostage situation where most women and girls are forced to self-censor, while suffering increasing harm due to the disappearance of free speech and safe spaces. It is, therefore, hardly surprising that, with all the political parties, institutions and businesses becoming hostile to women as a sex, handmaidens have become role models for success.

Looking to find their place in the gendered hierarchy, women can't be blamed for not wanting to be labelled "TERFs". Seeing the conditional nature of retaining any power as a woman - or indeed the conditional nature of women's rights - collaborating with the patriarchy is all that seems possible. This is why there is no shortage of women who are willing to throw other women under the bus and gain protection by signalling their allegiance to gender identity ideology.

Male rapists in female prisons

One area where gender identity ideology endangers women in particularly cruel ways, is with the placement of violent male offenders, who self-identify as women, into women's prisons.

A legal case from Texas, which attempted to stop this practice as early as 2016, described how male offenders, who were placed in housing units with women, were allowed to traumatise women with little, if any, consequences.

One particularly large male offender who has "assaulted at least two women--one because she did not give him a larger piece of cake and the second one in his housing area during a verbal disagreement", threatened to rape any woman who was housed with him because he did not want a cellmate.

Another "male inmate, with a penis, assaulted a female inmate in front of at least 100 women. He used vulgar language, threatening to "choke a b---h" with his penis to teach them a lesson."

None of these intact male inmates are mandated to take medication to prevent erections, and there is no sympathy for women who are being terrorised and assaulted. Instead, compassion and understanding are saved for these violent men, without regard for their attacks on women.

In their attempt to remove biological males from federal women's prisons, the State of Texas argued that placement of men into women's prisons is placing women in physical and emotional danger and that it "seems that the priority of the Defendants [United States of America] is to promote an ideology of transgender equal rights, bypassing Congress, while violating the constitutional rights of women in the community, as well as in women's prisons" (State of Texas vs United States of America, 2016).

Unfortunately, this practice continued, and two lawsuits have already been brought against the Illinois and California Departments of Correction by female inmates who claim to have been sexually assaulted by these men (Masterson, 2020; Southern, 2021).

Despite this, the ACLU has attempted to conceal the extent of the problem by filing a lawsuit against a woman who requested information from the Washington State Department of Corrections, about the number of male inmates housed in women's prisons (WoLF, 2021).

In the UK, male offenders who self-identified as women have been convicted of sexually assaulting female inmates (BBC, 2018; Brown, 2020). Despite this, when a female victim initiated a Judicial Review to stop the practice of placing male offenders into women's prisons, the Court ruled the MOJ's policy to house high-risk trans-identifying male inmates in female prisons was "capable of being operated lawfully". (FPFW, 2021).

In Ireland, violent and psychologically unstable men are terrorising women in Limerick women's prison (Law Society Gazette Ireland 2019; Women are Human, 2020).

It has now become clear that no amount of wilful endangerment of women by gender self-identification policies will be enough to make institutions across the Western world stop, and think, what it is they are enabling.

Escalating misogyny

Anyone who examines the issue of women's resistance to gender identity ideology, in good faith, will know that women aren't opposing gender self-identification because they are "paranoid fantasists" or "pearl-clutching prudes" who are spreading a "moral panic". They are regular women waking up to a dystopian nightmare in which any man can call himself a "trans woman" - or increasingly just "woman" - and get the state to help him victimise vulnerable women and girls with impunity.

This abusive male logic is masquerading as "trans rights activism", which seems to be paralysing institutions and stopping them from reviewing policies that are endangering women. Instead, women are forced to self-exclude from public life, healthcare and sport in order to avoid harm.

This stalemate is perpetuated by the general public's disbelief that all this is really happening, and the handmaidens reassurances that "trans women are women" and that there are no downsides to gender self-identification.

But something IS wrong.

Identifying *with* someone who isn't you is empathy. Identifying *as* someone who isn't you is identity theft. Men who claim they are women because they like/wear/do "women things" are seeing women through the eyes of an impostor, and their privilege to do this is defended with violence.

The art of misogyny

In 2018, a transactivist group Degenderettes Antifa Art was allowed to stage an exhibition celebrating violence against "TERFS" in San Francisco Public Library (Deep Green Resistance, 2018; Mag, 2018).

Shocking installations of white singlets with fake blood stains and slogans "I Punch TERFS" were exhibited alongside axes painted in trans colours, baseball bats wrapped in barbed wire, and riot shields that proclaimed "Die Cis Scum" - a slogan that was popularised in 2012 by trans-identifying male White Nationalist Char The Butcher.

The "artists" claimed that "TERF is an acronym for 'trans exclusionary (erasing) radical feminist', an oppressive belief-set that attempts to delegitimize trans women - not just theoretically, but by inducing suicide through internet harassment, public release of personal information, calls to employers and landlords, legal action and substantiated threats of death and physical harm - often directed against minors. It is possible that more trans deaths have occurred as a result of TERF harassment than by cis men homicides."

This unbridled display of aggression, coupled with unsubstantiated claims regarding suicide and violence against trans-identifying males, were designed to normalise and justify targeting of women who do not support the encroachment of men into women-only spaces.

Threat to child safeguarding

When trying to understand why transactivists are monstering feminists, we need to consider that women have always been at the forefront of defending not only the rights of women, and gender non-conforming adults, but also child safeguarding.

In 2018, one of the biggest LGBT+ media outlets published a story about an "openly gay" 3 year old boy. (Henderson, 2018). The article was immediately flagged up by readers as problematic. Being gay means being exclusively sexually attracted to members of the same sex. Children are not naturally sexually attracted to anyone, because they do not have sexual interests or an orientation prior to the commencement of puberty. Therefore, sexualised behaviours in children should always prompt an investigation into whether the child has been abused or exposed to sexually inappropriate content or behaviour. This understanding underlies child safeguarding. However, instead of apologising for projecting an adult sexuality onto a toddler, the LGBT+ media outlet claimed the criticism of their article was "homophobic abuse and bullying of a three year old child".

Gender identity ideology has also normalised "child drag queens" as a form of adult entertainment, and there are numerous videos and articles showing prepubescent boys performing in adult gay bars - sometimes having money thrown at them - being photographed with naked male drag queens, and being egged on by adults to make sexually explicit comments.

Combined with a push to lower the age of consent for medical gender reassignment procedures, with girls as young as 8 being given testosterone injections (Transgender Trend, 2019) and boys as young as 16 having surgical castration and vaginoplasty (Philby, 2012), it seems that transactivism isn't just driven by the desires of men to destroy women's sex-based rights. It also appears to be dismantling child safeguarding - a goal that is made easier by disempowering feminists.

Roll back on women's rights

Regardless of what anyone says, or orders us to think, men can't "identify as women" in any meaningful way. They can only identify as "trans" - whatever that means to them individually. To the rest of the society, they remain male. That's reality and as such, it should form the basis for policy and law, as well as social conventions.

Pronouns in the English language are sex-based and referring to a man as a "he" is accurate regardless of his "inner sense of gender identity". Calling a men "trans woman" or "she" is deliberately confusing and designed to create cognitive dissonance between what we say ("she") and what we see (male).

This is why I decided to no longer use the term "trans woman", but to use "man who claims to be a woman" or "trans-identifying male" instead.

My decision is not motivated by a desire to disrespect anyone's identity but by my strongly held belief that making a distinction between material reality and a male fantasy of womanhood is essential. Especially if we want to preserve the human rights of women and children, and combat the male violence inflicted on them.

I will also only use sex-appropriate pronouns. Out of respect - when that respect is warranted (and it's not when a man is abusive) - I'm prepared to use singular "they" or the person's name, but I'm committed to not using wrong sex pronouns even if I am being ordered to do so.

This brings me back to the handmaidens. While I understand their predicament, feminism is a journey from trying to comply with the demands of aggressive men, to finding courage to enforce strong boundaries with them. I no longer care how men will react when I say No. I am here to demand justice for victims of male violence, establish safety for women and children, and see repercussions for anyone in a position of power who has supported dangerous self-identification policies. The stakes are too high now, with children being abused and lied to, and women being harmed and disrespected in ways none of us could have ever imagined.

Bibliography

Moss, J. (2018). INTERVIEW: Maria MacLachlan on the GRA and the aftermath of her assault at Speaker's Corner. Feminist Current. https://www.feministcurrent.com/2018/06/21/interview-maria-maclauchlan-gra-aftermath-assault-speakers-corner/

State of Texas vs United States of America. (2016). United States District Court Northern District of Texas. Case 7:16-cv-00054-O. http://files.eqcf.org/wp-content/uploads/2017/02/102-Driever-et-al-Motion-for-PI.pdf

Masterson, M. (2020). Lawsuit: Female Prisoner Says She Was Raped by Transgender Inmate. WTTW. https://news.wttw.com/2020/02/19/lawsuit-female-prisoner-says-she-was-raped-transgender-inmate

Southern, K. California sued by Women's Liberation Front over transgender jail law that 'risks' safety. The Sunday Times. https://www.thetimes.co.uk/article/california-sued-by-womens-liberation-front-over-transgender-jail-law-that-risks-safety-jbn9gwrww

WoLF. (2021). ACLU Sues Private Citizen to Suppress Public Records Request in Washington State. https://www.prnewswire.com/news-releases/aclu-sues-private-citizen-to-suppress-public-records-request-in-washington-state-301268835.html

BBC. (2018). Trans inmate jailed for Wakefield prison sex offences. https://www.bbc.co.uk/news/uk-england-leeds-45825838

Brown, D. (2020). Seven sex attacks in women's jails by transgender convicts. The Sunday Times. https://www.thetimes.co.uk/article/seven-sex-attacks-in-womens-jails-by-transgender-convicts-cx9m8zqpg

FPFW. (2021). Transgender prison policy: judicial review ruling confirms trans rights do conflict with women's rights. Fair Play for Women. https://fairplayforwomen.com/transgender-prison-policy-judicial-review-ruling-confirms-trans-rights-do-conflict-with-womens-rights/

Law Society Gazette Ireland. (2019). Male-bodied transgender inmate housed with women. Gazette.ie. https://www.lawsociety.ie/gazette/top-stories/2019/10-october/male-bodied-transgender-inmate-housed-with-women-prisoners

Women are Human, (2020). Transgender Teen With Pattern of Violence Against Women "Anxious" to be Jailed With Women | Women Are Human.

https://www.womenarehuman.com/transgender-teen-charged-with-making-death-threats-against-two-individuals/

Deep Green Resistance. (2018). San Francisco Public Library Hosts Transgender "Art Exhibit" Featuring Weapons Intended to Kill Feminists. Medium. https://medium.com/@deepgreenresist/san-francisco-public-library-hosts-transgender-art-exhibit-featuring-weapons-intended-to-kill-3ccb82b34ab

Mag, G. (2018). San Francisco Public Library hosts transgender "art exhibit" featuring weapons intended to kill feminists. Gender Is Poison. https://genderispoison.wordpress.com/2018/04/27/san-francisco-public-library-hosts-transgender-art-exhibit-featuring-weapons-intended-to-kill-feminists/

Henderson, T. (2018). The Internet Is Head Over Heels for This Adorable, Openly Gay 3-Year-Old. Pride. https://webcache.googleusercontent.com/search?q=cache:TPTZO8ejjIcJ:https://www.pride.com/viral/2018/4/17/internet-head-over-heels-adorable-openly-gay-3-year-old+&cd=1&hl=en&ct=clnk&gl=ca

Transgender Trend. (2019). Johanna Olson-Kennedy and the US Gender Affirmative Approach. https://www.transgendertrend.com/johanna-olson-kennedy-gender-affirmative-approach/

Philby, Charlotte. (2012). How to deal with a transsexual teenage daughter (by a mother who knows). The Independent. https://www.independent.co.uk/life-style/health-and-families/features/how-deal-transexual-teenage-daughter-mother-who-knows-8329471.html

Chapter 12

The Myth of "Virtuous Paedophile" and Why P Should Not Be a Part of LGBT+

Pro-paedophilia activism has always been a problem on the internet. The dark corners where men who seek to abuse children meet and organise, are not rare in such a vast digital space. The little regulation that does exist can easily be evaded by locating servers in places where laws are lax or by relocating servers while the content remains live.

Paedophiles are notorious for operating in secret. They meet up - either in real life or online - to share fantasies, child sexual abuse (CSA) content and tips on how to procure victims. They also traffic children away from prying eyes.

Paedophiles are relentless in trying to legitimise their proclivities and are experts in the grooming of adults, particularly those in positions of power or authority such as parents, therapists, prison staff and even politicians.

Throughout history, paedophiles have found ways to legitimise their abuse. Here are a few examples:

- Pederasty in Ancient Greece, which allowed adult men to sexually enslave and exploit boys. (The Free Library, 2014)
- "Bachabaze" in Afghanistan, which allows wealthy men to sexually abuse boy dancers as young as 12 (Quobil, 2010)
- Rape of boys by adult warriors as an initiation ritual of the Sambia tribe in Papua New Guinea (Anderson, 2018)
- UK government-sanctioned Paedophile Information Exchange (De Castella & Heyden, 2014)
- Berlin authorities deliberately placing homeless children with known paedophiles, under the assumption that these child molesters would be "ideal foster parents" (Deutsche Welle, 2020)
- The North American Man-Boy Love Association (NAMBLA), which still campaigns to allow paedophiles to sexually exploit children (DeYoung, 1989)
- Child abusers such as priests, politicians and celebrities, who were not only tolerated but were actively protected by the authorities and those around them (Laville et al, 2013).

Paedophilia, or a sexual disorder in which an adult, or older adolescent, is primarily or exclusively sexually attracted to prepubescent children, is found almost exclusively in men. Therefore, it is unsurprising that paedophilia has been particularly pernicious and difficult to stamp out. We live in a patriarchy, which prioritises male sexual desires and other privileges above all else. Enabling men with sexual perversions is part and parcel of living in such a system.

One of the enduring myths about paedophilia is that it is a "sexual orientation like any other". On this basis, some have argued that paedophilia should be "destigmatised" and that paedophiles should be included under the LGBT+ umbrella.

Is paedophilia a sexual orientation?

Paedophiles, just like anyone else, already have a sexual orientation depending on whether they are sexually attracted to members of the same sex (homosexual), opposite sex (heterosexual) or both sexes (bisexual). Sexual orientation, by itself, is not abusive. What is abusive is when sexual activity is inflicted on someone who either didn't, or couldn't, consent.

One of the primary purposes of sexual activity is sexual reproduction, which occurs between males and females. This is why heterosexual orientation is the most common. However, because there are other benefits to sexual intercourse besides reproduction - such as pleasure and bonding - homosexuality and bisexuality, are also natural, albeit minority, sexual orientations.

It needs to be said that sexual coercion in humans, like in all primates, is not uncommon. To mitigate this, some primates have evolved to require female orgasm for conception. In this way, females ensure that they are in charge of mate selection, even when stronger males rape them. Unfortunately, this is not the case in humans and, throughout history, men have been able to sexually coerce or trick women and girls into sexual intercourse, in order to pass on their genes.

In this era of overpopulation, it is easy to forget how long humans have struggled to produce enough offspring to overcome high mortality rates. However, the argument that rape - by violence or deception - is a good method to ensure the survival of the human species has never been convincing.

Women, like men, are born with a biological imperative to procreate and they are instinctively equipped to choose males that have a chance of producing the fittest offspring, either due to superior/compatible genetics or a willingness to help raise the young. Taking this choice away from a woman undermines the basic process of mate selection and ultimately works against the survival of the species.

Selfish males who sexually coerce women seldom make good fathers and providers. Their violence, neglect, and abandonment create significant psychological and physical trauma, which is passed on to the next generation, creating a cycle of despair and destructiveness.

Therefore, while our patriarchal culture assumes that the way our society had developed in the context of endemic male violence must have been "for the best", it is equally if not more likely that the effects of this (such as neglect, abandonment and violence directed at women and children) has created a society stuck in a self-perpetuating cycle of destructiveness.

Paedophilia is even further removed from a sane evolutionary strategy than the rape of women is, because it serves no biological imperative whatsoever. Prepubescent children can neither produce offspring nor cope with being sexually exploited by adults. They, overwhelmingly, suffer in such encounters and they and their caregivers need to be tricked, deceived and coerced to submit to the abusers. Even more than adult rape, child sexual abuse traumatises and harms the victims, and it causes severe physical and psychological injuries that are rarely seen in any other context. Therefore, while it's hard to comprehend how a man can derive pleasure from rape, it is even more incomprehensible how he can find pleasure in sexually assaulting a defenceless child.

One aspect that could possibly be explored is the fact that research suggests rapists and paedophiles are plagued by intrusive sexual abuse fantasies and strong, almost irresistible, compulsions to act on them. The discrepancy between paedophiles who seek treatment before they offend, and the sheer number of child sexual abuse victims, makes it unlikely, however, that obsessions and compulsions alone are the salient feature of paedophilia. Instead, I see sexual sadism, lack of empathy and narcissistic entitlement as core drivers, which makes paedophilia a criminal predisposition rather than a sexual orientation.

Child sex dolls and the myth of the "virtuous paedophile"

In 2019, one of the biggest platforms where pro-paedophilia activism has thrived - Tumblr - introduced new rules regarding sexually explicit content. This caused a mass migration of paedophiles, or MAPs ("minor attracted persons"), to Twitter and other social media platforms. Familiar with the old trope of a violent and obviously creepy paedophile, the readers were suddenly faced with well-groomed images of the "virtuous paedophile", a tortured and conflicted man who claims to have never harmed a child and who is begging society to allow him to pacify his intrusive, unwanted child abuse fantasies in "safer" ways. These ways never seem to include voluntary incarceration or chemical castration. Instead, these men and their enablers are proposing online support groups for paedophiles, unfettered access to child sex dolls and child sexual abuse content, and the inclusion of paedophiles into the LGBT+ community.

It's not just the average, uninformed person who risks falling for the paedophile sob story. Paedophile rights are being championed by some reputable professionals, who may be very pleasant and empathetic when discussing the difficult predicament paedophiles find themselves in, but are quick to accuse women who question them, of "moral panic" and "ideologically driven rants" (Harper, 2018).

In my discussions with "virtuous paedophile" activists, I have found that they angrily demand citations which prove that "virtuous" paedophiles, child abuse images and child sex dolls are harmful to children. When the evidence is provided (Meridian, et al., 2011; Pessimism about pedophilia. There is no cure, so the focus is on protecting children, 2010; Brown & Shelling, 2019), they either refuse to believe it, dismiss the source or shift the goalposts, never answering difficult questions that would make most people stop and consider the pitfalls of what they're promoting.

"Virtuous paedophile" advocates also like to assert their authority and claim that "most therapists agree with them" (which is demonstrably untrue), that they are "entirely free of bias" (yeah, right) and that they should be the sole authority in conversations about the dangerousness of paedophiles. In contrast to their assertions, I have found them to be professionally disinterested in discussing the harms child sexual abuse inflicts on victims. They have no answer, either, for the fact that pornography and child sexual abuse images have existed for centuries, and that this has done nothing to reduce the numbers of children who are being sexually exploited by adults, which remains at endemic levels throughout the world.

The sense I got was that they believed they were pioneers and on the cutting edge of their fields, while their opponents were conservative and ignorant.

In reality, the idea that paedophiles should be enabled to satisfy their urges in "safer" ways isn't revolutionary at all. The belief that a man not being able to orgasm in whatever way he wants is a tragedy, and something - no matter how drastic - must be done about it, is in fact the bread and butter of male supremacy. To this end, men have created prostitution, pornography, sex dolls and even the oppression of women, which includes an expectation that women will do whatever it takes to satisfy male sexual urges, and take responsibility for male sexual offending.

This approach has the same effect on eradicating rape and child sexual abuse as pouring gasoline has on putting out a fire. It gives people an opportunity to say that they did something, even if they have to avert their eyes from the results of their intervention.

Paedophilia treatment programmes

There is an argument for scientific curiosity in all this, of course. Clinicians have vowed to try and help anyone who is suffering, regardless of who, or what, they are and a degree of empathy is warranted even for those who are a threat to others, because they did not ask to be "born this way".

I might think that allowing paedophiles to use child sex dolls for practice runs of their molestation fantasies is a supremely stupid and dangerous idea, but there is a way to scientifically interrogate that hypothesis. For example, by doing a study on incarcerated paedophiles, who would be given supervised access to child sex dolls so that the effect on their fantasies and risk could be assessed in a controlled environment and without endangering children. Experimentation on prisoners might be prohibited for all kinds of ethical reasons, but the alternative -

free sale of child sex dolls - is even more unethical, considering the potential harms.

So far, and not for the lack of trying, paedophilia is considered incurable and treatments that focus on harm prevention, such as chemical castration, incarceration and supervision in the community, work best to reduce risk to children.

On the other hand, group therapy for sex offenders has shown to increase that risk.

In the UK, the Ministry of Justice suspended the Core Sex Offender Treatment Programme (SOTP) in 2017, after it was shown that it led to more reoffending. Offering group therapy and psychological help to high risk sex offenders, whilst a reasonable idea on the surface, showed that "group treatment may 'normalise' individuals' behaviour. When stories are shared, their behaviour may not be seen as wrong or different; or at worst, contacts and sources associated with sexual offending may be shared." (Casciani, 2017)

There might be some modest evidence for the benefit of various psychotherapies such as psychoanalysis, cognitive-behavioural therapy, aversion therapy or even attempts to redirect the sexual focus of paedophiles to more appropriate targets, such as adult women. I don't see how inflicting men who are aroused by sexually abusing non-consenting partners, onto women who are already vulnerable to physical and sexual abuse by men, is safe or progressive at all. Furthermore, I am concerned that some paedophile treatment centres are enabling abusers, due to policies to not report clients who disclose a past history of abusing children, and even in cases of clients disclosing current plans to harm a child, contacting authorities is seen as the last resort (Smith, 2021).

If our aim is to reduce harm to children, and free

paedophiles from the fantasies and compulsions that drive them to sexually abuse children, it is hardly an unreasonable leap of logic to say it is dangerous to encourage them to organise via online clubs and support groups, where they can share their fantasies, experiences and child abuse images. Indeed, doing this and then providing them with extremely realistic looking, yet completely passive and compliant, child sex dolls, would in all probability increase, rather than decrease, their likelihood of offending.

Does P belong in LGBTQ+?

Some paedophiles are low IQ individuals who suffer from sexual immaturity and poor impulse control. Others are intelligent and have made it their life's work to find a way to make their fantasies a reality, and to do it without getting caught. When they are caught grooming, molesting, or using child abuse images, they protest their innocence despite all evidence to the contrary, claiming to be falsely accused and painting their victims as perpetrators. They also groom adults into ignoring red flags, which enables them to abuse children more easily.

Throughout history, paedophiles have taken advantage of the laws that allow men to gain unrestricted access to children - such as in the context of marriage, adoption, fostering and servitude.

When applying for jobs, paedophiles typically don't disclose their fantasies about child molestation or their history of offending, not because they "fear discrimination" but because they fear being denied access to children.

Any paedophile who has insight into the potential dangerousness of his fantasies, and the compulsion to translate them into real-life acts, wouldn't apply for a job that brings him into close contact with children in the first place. However, despite all the talk about "virtuous" and "non-offending" paedophiles and ongoing attempts to reduce their risk of offending using various psychotherapies, many pedophiles gravitate toward professions that give them a cloak of respectability and access to children, such as judges, doctors, teachers, priests, social workers, and charity sector employees.

This is such a common way for paedophiles to procure victims that society has had to develop safeguarding frameworks in order to prevent anyone with paedophilic proclivities from working with children.

Imagine now if paedophiles were added to the LGBTQ+ rainbow and given the same rights and protections as gay, lesbian, bisexual and trans-identifying people. For paedophiles, marriage equality means ability to marry children. Anti-discrimination employment laws would make refusing to employ a paedophile in a kindergarten a case of "discrimination based on sexual orientation". Objecting to paedophilic proclivities could become a "hate crime" called "paedophobia".

Pro-paedophilia activists also claim that anyone who opposes adults sexually exploiting children is being "ageist" and "denying children autonomy". They assert that "not all sex with children is harmful", and "if no harm has occurred then adults having sex with children should be legal". These claims go hand in hand with portraying paedophiles as "misunderstood" and turning a blind eye to the coercive tactics they use to gaslight and discredit their victims.

The history of pro-paedophilia activism among postmodern theorists, who have birthed the "queer" and "gender identity" movements, has also led to the re-vitalisation of the pro-paedophilia movement. In a brilliant four-part series, a feminist historian known on social media as Dr EM, explored how postmodernists and queer theorists have variously supported lowering or abolishing the age of consent, legitimising "consensual sex" between adults and minors and the legalisation of child abuse images (Dr EM, 2019)

Queer theory, which is rooted in the transgression of boundaries, relativisation of evidence and the acceptance of self-identification "without exception", has eroded existing safeguards. Children are being given puberty blockers, which are designed to arrest their development in the pre-pubertal stage, while institutions are telling us "when people tell you who they are believe them", which includes men claiming to be women or even little girls (James, 2015). Sexual fetishes and sexually explicit content have been embraced during ostensibly child-friendly Pride parades. Incidents, such an employee of a child charity making rubber fetish videos at work, are now more likely to result in support than sanction from the employer (Bartosch, 2019).

With the LGBTQ+ movement already steeped in queer theory, the addition of paedophiles is unlikely to bode well for the safety and rights of children. A cursory glance at the pro-paedophilia activism content online, illustrates this in chilling detail.

Paedophile manifesto

In 2018, Dr EM posted an insightful thread on twitter, analysing an anonymous Paedophile Manifesto titled "After The Fall: A Beginner's Guide to Destroying Pedophobia in the 21st Century". (Dr EM, 2018; Anonymous, 2015).

This manifesto is hosted on "Boy Wiki", which describes itself as "an exciting opportunity for us, as boylovers, to record and preserve our own history, culture, and heritage. If it's of interest to boylovers, it belongs on BoyWiki, so feel free to explore what we have to offer: you can read anything on the site without signing up, and most entries are freely redistributable under the terms of the GNU Free Documentation License" (Boy Wiki, 2015).

In this manifesto, pro-paedophilia activists demonstrate various strategies - including forced teaming of their cause with LGB activism - they intend to use to groom and subvert society and its laws and norms.

I will now include some quotes from this document, to illustrate just how detailed and well thought-out these sinister strategies are. All emphasis in italics is mine.

From the outset, the manifesto likens paedophilia to same-sex attraction, claiming that, "as late as the 1970s adult-child relationships were no more controversial than same-sex ones" and they blame "conservative administrations" and "sex-negative radical feminists" for "restrictive bills that liken a serious crime (the abuse, rape and torture of children) to something completely harmless (nude photos)".

They use linguistic sleight of hand to reframe the rational fear of paedophiles as "pedophobia" - by which they mean an "irrational fear or hatred of child sexuality" - and claim that "while pedophilia is natural, independently appearing in several modern and ancient societies across the world, pedophobia isn't".

They seek to expose children to adult sexual behaviour by creating a so-called "sex-positive society" where "clothes become the exception, not the rule because the only way to destigmatise the genitals is through frequent social nudity". Once nudity is normalised, pro-paedophilia activists propose "adding another body" to normalise sexual activity in public. "The message needs to be pushed" they say "that *you are every part of you, and every part is normal*. It is ok to touch yourself or others in public (if you get the permission, of course!)."

They refer to this as a "cascading effect of loosening boundaries" which should eventually lead one "to respond to someone playing with themselves in the same way you would if you saw them eating a hamburger".

In order to safeguard this "fragile" cascade, the manifesto instructs activists to encourage public support for those who go nude by referring to them as *"brave"* and *"bold"*, and they believe that "social media and advertising campaigns will play a large part in the push to make nudity normal".

However, ubiquitous nudism is not the endgame.

In the section titled "Strategies For Acceptance: Psychological" the author(s) propose a slow "boiling a frog" method to normalising paedophilia:

"We must seek realistic, common-sense reforms. On the surface, our appeal isn't radical at all: Just treat sex like we treat any other activity, and require parental consent for children to engage in it. If something happens or the child catches an STD, we can hold the parents (and the one who transmitted it) liable...*At the end of the day, what happens should be the child's choice because it's their body.*"

"But let's not get ahead of ourselves. We mustn't shock and repel the public with the mental imagery of kind sex in the beginning of our campaign. Instead, *wherever possible, pedosexuality must be reduced to an abstract question and vague feelings of love, kindness and nurturing.*"

The word "kind" references the German word "kinder," i.e. child. Therefore, the phrase "kind sex" refers to "child sex" while simultaneously utilising the meaning of the words "kind" and "kindness" in the English language.

The manifesto goes on to describe the process of grooming in disturbing detail:

"Dull the public sense of panic and fear whenever the subject of children and sexuality comes up. The principle behind this is clear. Any behaviour becomes more acceptable the more people talk about it or see their friends talking about it. This is accomplished by a large groundswell of open and furtive talk about pedosexuality in a natural or positive way....A chain reaction occurs where more and more people come out. Bring up your sexual orientation as much as possible in a humorous manner to break the ice...Discussion moves the idea from 'unthinkable' to 'controversial' in the Overton Window, and that's one step toward 'normal'."

They advocate for widespread media campaigns about paedophile rights:

"Where you talk is important. Internet comment sections are helpful, but they aren't places to have a debate...Better places to speak include local newspapers, magazines and television. While you won't be able to openly support pedosexuality at first, you can support sex-positive and pro-nudity initiatives in your area."

And they propose to exhaust the population as well as shame them about not being progressive enough:

"The main point is to talk about kindness until the issue becomes thoroughly exhausting. People should come to view being kind the same way they do liking a certain flavor of ice cream. The process of desensitization can be sped up by making comments which allude to the matter being settled when someone very emotive appears. *Dude, why do you care so much? It's just sex.*"

"(In response to 'children can't consent') 'I'm so tired of this stupid myth still being spread around' (link to a better source or explanation). *'You're behind the times.* Nobody cares anymore.'"

Paedophiles are also advised to operate in groups, in order to give an illusion of mass support:

"Never go alone during desensitization efforts. Always bring backup. There's nothing worse than being the only person in a comment section battling against hordes of bigots. If you see someone trying to fight ignorance online, don't just stand there, help them out!'"

"Desensitization is important in real life too. You have to come out and be completely normal. If you live among straights in peace, while they might find you annoying they will eventually get used to you. Flooding culture in a wave of kind-positive advertising and media inevitably leads to changes in social values."

They refer to the process of guilt-tripping, shaming and ostracising those who oppose child sexual abuse, as "jamming":

"We want to shut down the thought process which leads to pedophobic remarks in the first place. Most of us know that people make those tough-guy statements for a quick shot of self-righteousness or social approval. 'Jamming' implies the addition of a second, mutually exclusive emotion. Guilt. Most people feel shame when they make a lame joke or say something deemed socially unacceptable. With enough jamming, the pedophobe's mental state can be worn down to meagre acceptance."

"The easiest way to 'jam' is to call out people who say prejudicial things. Tell them it's not okay, make videos about it online. On youtube in particular, take the worst comments, do dramatic readings and laugh at them. When people see the ingroup rejecting their mean-spirited comments, most will stop saying them. Remember how calling things 'gay' used to be cool? Let's do that for us."

Young and hip people are an essential part of this strategy. They are to be manipulated to "call out the bigots":

"Jamming is even more effective when a bigot sees people like him disapproving of his statement. If our target audience is young, teenage progressives, then pictures and videos must be made of hipsters ridiculing people making fun of kinds. If our target is parents, show parents AND children correcting them."

Anyone opposed to child sexual abuse is to be ostracised:

"All we have to do is make pedophobes believe that they are unpopular. Jamming works by defining the limits of acceptable speech and shifting them. *By repeatedly labelling opposition 'pedophobes' or 'anti-sex', a hostile environment is created for pedophobic speech.*"

Pro-paedophilia activists aim to recruit "true allies" who would help them normalise paedophilia:

"Long term, we are safest if we sincerely 'convert' those against us into true 'allies'. We can spread stories of confessions, testimonials and other straights who 'evolved' their views on pedosexuality."

They hope to achieve this using a media strategy to liken their opponents to "racists", while portraying paedophiles as "victims":

"The ultimate reward for prejudice is a feeling of self-righteousness and acceptance from a bigot's 'crowd'. Ads that conflict with this self-image as a well-liked person lead to guilt - cancelling out this reward. For this reason, *pedophobic bigots must be treated in the media as crude loudmouths and assholes who use all kinds of slurs long-gone ('nigger', 'fag', 'kike', 'lynching').*"

"We can depict kinds experiencing terrible suffering as a direct result of his pedophobia - the kind most reasonable people would be ashamed to cause. Link pedo-shaming to all kinds of disliked attributes. Show pedophobes being hated, shunned and criticized."

In the section titled "Strategies For Acceptance: Social" pro-paedophilia activists are encouraged to:

Come out

"You need to come out and encourage others to do so, especially if you haven't 'offended' yet. Start saving money for a 'coming out fund' just in case you get fired. Organise a massive 'coming out day' where large groups of kinds agree to make coming-out videos and release them on youtube at the same time...Hiding only helps further oppression."

Portray kinds as victims

"Kinds must be portrayed as victims of nature, not people who willingly choose their attraction. Who would actually choose to be a part of the world's most hated group anyway? As far as you know, you were born kind and you cannot change it."

Liken therapy for paedophiles to conversion therapy

"Efforts at 'therapy' must be considered harmful and damaging to your identity. Frequently compare it to bleaching blacks or reformation camps."

"By appearing as victims, the majority is instinctively inclined to protect and defend."

Give allies a just cause

"You need a 'just cause', and in your case plain legal equality leaves too much to be desired since children can never have all the legal rights of an adult. A just cause answers the question 'I'm not one of you, so why should I care?'"

Force-team paedophilia activism with other, more socially acceptable activism

"Our causes are sex-positivity, anti-ageism, bodily autonomy and the right to privacy. The government shouldn't have the

authority to tell people what they can and can't do inside the bedroom or dictate how parents must raise their children. If no physical or emotional harm is being done, there is no excuse to ban an activity."

"You also have an excellent just cause in religious liberty; *childhood innocence and harmfulness of sex are religious beliefs you shouldn't be forced to believe.* Morality should never be backed by legislation."

Rewrite history

"Make kinds look good."

"We know this trick is old as dirt, but kinds must also be portrayed as pillars of society. *Using historical figures is excellent because they are no longer living and can't sue. Anyone who's even believed to have had the slightest attraction to or relationship with someone under 18 will be considered a pedosexual for our purposes.* Elvis anyone? We understand that that's not the medical definition, but confusing social and medical definition is actually helpful in this case."

"Make pedophobes look bad."

"At a later stage of the media campaign for kind rights - long after other ads have become commonplace - it'll be time to get tough with remaining pedo-bashers."

"The public should be shown images of ranting pedophobes whose secondary traits and beliefs disgust middle America. These images might include: the Ku Klux Klan demanding that kinds be burned alive or castrated; bigoted southern ministers drooling with hysterical hatred to a degree that looks both comical and deranged; menacing punks, thugs and convicts speaking cooly about the 'pedos' they have killed or would like to kill; a tour of Nazi concentration camps where kinds were tortured and gassed."

"*Loudly and constantly compare pedophobic bigots to segre-*

gationists, WBC klansmen, hypocrites and gay-bashers. Make the contrast clear: Either you're for social tolerance, or you're for gruesome violence."

* * *

Reading this manifesto, I was struck by how much it mirrors the arguments transactivists use to enable men who claim to be women to enter female prisons, rape crisis shelters, women's sports, and women's toilets.

Feminists have been fighting this trend in law, with ethics and logic. However, it has been an uphill battle because many bend over backwards to prioritise male needs for sexual gratification and validation over the safety of women and children. Now we have a new contender in the fight - paedophiles and their enablers.

Worst of all is the misogyny responsible for society routinely dismissing women's safeguarding concerns while buying into bad faith arguments which pro-paedophilia activists assert with impunity. For example, just because there are some paedophiles who haven't, allegedly, molested a child yet, doesn't mean that they haven't abused children by proxy, by using child abuse images. I can't see how anyone can prove that a paedophile is "virtuous" or "non-offending". The only thing that can be proven is the absence of a conviction, and that really doesn't count for much, not when child safety from sexual abuse is at stake.

Therefore, my position is that nurturing the myth of a "virtuous paedophile", facilitating their access to child sex dolls and giving paedophiles the same rights as other members of LGBTQ+ community, would not only normalise child molestation and put state power behind paedophile grooming tactics, it would further dismantle painstakingly built safeguarding frameworks. Additionally, it would make it near impossible for victims to discuss what was being done to them, without them being accused of "bigotry" and "pedophobia". Instead of racing to embrace any and all social transgression in the name of progress, tolerance and inclusivity, we need to strengthen the existing laws that prevent paedophiles from manipulating their way into easier access to victims.

Bibliography

The Free Library. (2014). Sex between Men and Boys in Classical Greece: Was It Education for Citizenship or Child Abuse?. (n.d.) https://www.thefreelibrary.com/Sex+between+Men+and+Boys+in+Classical+Greece%3a+Was+It+Education+for...-a072684381

Quobil, R. (2010). The sexually abused dancing boys of Afghanistan. BBC. https://www.bbc.co.uk/news/world-south-asia-11217772

Anderson, C. (2018) 'Not all sex involving children is abuse': Gay Rights activist Peter Tatchell is forced to deny 'advocating paedophilia' after 1997 letter about Papua New Guinea tribes emerges. Mail Online. https://www.dailymail.co.uk/news/article-6374467/Peter-Tatchell-forced-deny-advocating-paedophilia-1997-letter.html

De Castella, T. Heyden, T. (2014) How did the pro-paedophile group PIE exist openly for 10 years? BBC News. https://www.bbc.co.uk/news/magazine-26352378

Deutsche Welle. (2020) Berlin authorities placed children with pedophiles for 30 years. https://www.dw.com/en/berlin-authorities-placed-children-with-pedophiles-for-30-years/a-53814208

DeYoung, M. (1989) World According to NAMBLA: Accounting for Deviance. Journal of Sociology and Social Welfare Volume: 16 Issue: 1 Dated: (March 1989) Pages: 111-126. https://www.ojp.gov/ncjrs/virtual-library/abstracts/world-according-nambla-accounting-deviance

Laville, S. Addley, E. Halliday, J (2013). Police errors left Jimmy Savile free to 'groom the nation'. The Guardian. https://www.theguardian.com/uk/2013/jan/11/jimmy-savile-police-report

Harper, C. (2018). Let's Talk About Sex (Dolls). Medium. https://medium.com/craig-harper-essays/lets-talk-about-sex-dolls-50f9be2e6198

Meridian, H.L. Curtis, C. Thakker, J. Wilson, N. Boer, D.P. (2011). The three dimensions of online child pornography offending. Journal of Sexual Aggression. DOI:10.1080/13552600.2011.611898. https://eprints.lincoln.ac.uk/id/eprint/4838/1/3dimensions_final.pdf

Pessimism about pedophilia. There is no cure, so the focus is on protecting children. Harv Ment Health Lett. 2010 Jul;27(1):1-3. PMID: 20812410. https://pubmed.ncbi.nlm.nih.gov/20812410/ full text available on http://adam.curry.com/art/1561299099_kCYxfaNb.html and https://web.archive.

org/web/20220816224232/http://adam.curry.com/art/1561299099_kCYxfaNb.html

Brown, R. Shelling, J. (2019). Exploring the implications of child sex dolls. Trends & issues in crime and criminal justice no. 570. Canberra: Australian Institute of Criminology. https://www.aic.gov.au/publications/tandi/tandi570

Casciani, D. (2017). Sex offender treatment in prison led to more offending. BBC News. https://www.bbc.co.uk/news/uk-40460637

Smith, J. M. (2021). Can a Radical Treatment for Paedophilia Work Outside of Germany? Science Wire. https://science.thewire.in/health/can-a-radical-treatment-for-paedophilia-work-outside-of-germany/

Dr EM. (2019). The Trojan Unicorn: Queer Theory and Paedophilia, Part I. Uncommonground Media. https://uncommongroundmedia.com/the-trojan-unicorn-queer-theory-and-paedophilia-part-i-dr-em/

James, E. (2015). 'I've gone back to being a child': Husband and father-of-seven, 52, leaves his wife and kids to live as a transgender SIX-YEAR-OLD girl named Stefonknee. Mail Online. https://www.dailymail.co.uk/femail/article-3356084/I-ve-gone-child-Husband-father-seven-52-leaves-wife-kids-live-transgender-SIX-YEAR-OLD-girl-named-Stefonknee.html

Bartosch, J. (2019). NSPCC Employee Films Himself Masturbating at Work. Uncommon Ground Media. https://uncommongroundmedia.com/nspcc-employee-films-himself-masturbating-at-work/

Dr EM. (2018). Analysis of Paedophile Manifesto. https://mobile.twitter.com/PankhurstEM/status/991258043366232064

Anonymous (2015). After The Fall: A Beginner's Guide to Destroying Pedophobia in the 21st Century. https://archive.ph/7c6pR

BoyWiki (2015). (Boylove Essays) - After The Fall: A Beginner's Guide to Destroying Pedophobia in the 21st Century. https://www.boywiki.org/en/(Boylove_Essays)_-_After_The_Fall:_A_Beginner's_Guide_to_Destroying_Pedophobia_in_the_21st_Century

Chapter 13

CASE STUDY 3 - Deny, Attack, Reverse Victim and Offender (DARVO)

There is no polite way to say this - transactivism has used psychological manipulation through methods such as emotional blackmail, false suicide statistics and gaslighting, to achieve many of its goals.

For example, the transactivists campaign for self-declared gender identity to replace biological sex in all institutional policies, including prisons. As they believe in "trans women are women" and "acceptance without exception", they see nothing wrong with allowing male rapists who "self-identify as women" to be housed in female prisons.

When feminists present evidence that some of these men attack and rape women inmates, transactivists gaslight them. They **D**eny that this happens and **A**ccuse female inmates of lying and the feminists of being "transphobic bigots" who want to deny "trans women" their human rights. By doing this, they **R**everse the **V**ictim and **O**ffender (**DARVO**).

DARVO has been so successful at convincing institutions that the trans-identifying men are more real, more suffering and more deserving victims than women, that allowing such men into women-only spaces - including rape crisis shelters, prisons and hospital wards - has become commonplace. What's more, these men have been elevated to a blameless, almost sacred caste that must never be challenged, their every whim and demand catered to by institutions and businesses, while women who object have been persecuted, maligned and ignored.

I'm not suggesting that everyone who promotes gender self-identification - or profits from it - is an abuser. However, many proponents of this ideology have learned to use DARVO to force society to comply with their unreasonable demands. The outcome of this is a horrible climate of "no debate" in which ongoing harm to women and children can neither be acknowledged nor discussed in good faith.

I believe that one way out of this predicament is to educate as many people as possible about DARVO - what it looks like and what it can achieve. To this end, I would like to present a case I encountered in my clinical practice, followed by a discussion of how this behavioural pattern has become a political strategy. I hope this rather extreme example will help others to recognise this particular behaviour when they encounter it.

Case study

One evening, I was called to the Accident and Emergency Department to assess a middle-aged senior manager following an insulin overdose. The insulin belonged to his 13 year old niece, who he was accused of molesting.

The patient was a tall, well-groomed man who looked like he had recently lost a lot of weight. He had dark circles under his eyes, a tormented expression on his face and he appeared too upset to talk.

Due to fluctuating blood glucose levels, he was initially admitted to a medical ward. A couple of days later when his condition stabilised, he was transferred to psychiatry.

The handover from the medical team indicated that this "poor man" had most likely been falsely accused. He confided in several staff members about being worried his niece had been abused by another man and appeared devastated that she had "mistakenly" accused him instead.

He proceeded to settle well on 1:1 suicide watch, and he received a lot of care and attention from the nurses. Then the police came to inform him that he had been charged with sexually abusing his niece.

Over the next few days, it transpired that the stories he told us were false. His niece, an insulin-dependent diabetic, had been spending after-school afternoons at her uncle's house. The family thought they were close until she admitted to her mother that her uncle was molesting her. The police were in receipt of physical and photo evidence that corroborated her testimony.

When our patient realised that the game was up, his demeanour changed. We watched his meek, grieving face morph into an angry scowl. The previously gentle, measured words became spitting hisses. The story about his niece changed too. You see, she was in fact a "whore and a liar". She had "come on to him" and "got angry when he rejected her".

What followed was a three-month long nightmare on the ward. This upstanding, wealthy pillar of the community became a furious and vindictive paedophile. He accused multiple nurses of molesting him, and while the filth that was coming out of his mouth is unrepeatable, suffice it to say that his misogyny, hatred and projection were extraordinary.

Whenever he became stable enough to be discharged back home to await trial, he would take another overdose, timing the call to the ambulance perfectly, so that he was always rescued in time.

He continued to blame his niece for falsely accusing him. However, he delighted in showing some staff that he was lying. He would sob as he repeated his sad tale to anyone who would listen and then turn around and smirk at us. As his lies and overdoses escalated, he was diagnosed with Passive Aggressive Personality Disorder, and due to a high suicide risk, he was committed under the Mental Health Act.

I will never forget his first Mental Health Review Board meeting, where he had the opportunity to contest his involuntary admission. My male boss went with me to back me up, knowing it would be hard for me to cope with this patient's misogynistic abuse on my own. The patient was physically imposing, and he would scowl, spit and unleash a torrent of lies and abuse at any opportunity. He was articulate, convincing, and very intimidating.

In a ten minute rant that felt more like two hours, he accused all of us of being paedophiles and child molesters. He fabricated numerous incidents including medication errors, incompetence on the doctors' part and stories of nurses injecting themselves with drugs and having sex with other patients - something that I knew for a fact was not true because I visited the ward often, and unpredictably, at all hours of day and night. The intensity of his anger and the ease and elaborate nature of his lies was so shocking, that by the end of his allotted time the review board were speechless.

This was the first time I had witnessed full-blown DARVO, and I just kept thanking my lucky stars that I was seeing it in a controlled environment. Imagine how this would have played out without security close by and if everyone wasn't fully aware of the iron-clad evidence against him.

Soon afterwards, he was transferred to a high security psychiatric unit and I never saw him again. Despite the passage of time, however, I am still somewhat traumatised for witnessing it. On the positive side, I have found this experience very instructive and I have never lost the ability to recognise this type of behaviour.

Discussion

I think that DARVO works so well for three reasons. Firstly, it obscures and confuses the issues in abusive situations. No sooner does a rape victim identify her abuser than she is labeled a liar or accused of seducing the alleged rapist and trying to ruin his life. This instantly puts the onus on the victim to prove that she is not, in fact, the actual abuser. By doing this, the abuser diverts attention from his wrongdoing which helps him to escape the consequences of his actions.

Secondly, abusers are experienced liars, and they rarely put the brakes on their behaviour. The more threatened they are, the bigger their lies become, and they tell them with such conviction that an ordinary, honest person has no way of beating them at their own game.

Thirdly, most of us are afraid to challenge abusers. When we witness someone being abused, we instinctively avert our eyes and tell ourselves that the victim must have done something to deserve it. We do this so that we can avoid confrontation with the abuser, who may be dangerous to us, as well. In turn, anyone who feels compelled to stand up for the victim knows that they will probably be the only ones doing it, as the onlookers avoid getting involved or even side with the abuser to protect themselves.

Abusers are aware of this dynamic and take full advantage of it by turning any challenge to their behaviour into a "you are either with me or against me" game. This serves to isolate the victim. The victim is now the odd one out, an inconvenience at best and a threat at worst, while the abuser has all the support.

Evidence and calm discussion are powerless against DARVO - at least for a while. Eventually, abusers lose control, the mask slips, and they get exposed. By then, it's often too late. The extended period of gaslighting and the reversing of victim and offender has bought time for systems to be put in place to benefit the abuser.

In criminal proceedings, abusers use DARVO to generate enough reasonable doubt to convince the judge and jury they should acquit them. Or they wage extended DARVO campaigns in family courts, which can leave their spouses destitute and their children traumatised. The mere threat of this is often enough to intimidate victims into shrinking away from seeking justice or holding their abusers to account.

Ultimately, DARVO is a tactic that carries enormous potential gains for the abuser while having few risks. If DARVO doesn't work out the way it was intended - for example, the irrefutable proof is provided, and authorities act to stop the abuser - the society will shrug their shoulders and say, "well, he is an abuser, what did you expect?". If it does work, the abuser wins, and the lives of his victim - and anyone who attempted to help her - are ruined.

Transactivist DARVO

The transactivist utilisation of DARVO becomes obvious when they respond to concerns that sexual predators would use gender self-identification laws to gain access to victims. They have no compunction in comparing women who fight for sex-based rights and child safeguarding, such as JK Rowling, to prolific child molesters, such as Jimmy Saville. They claim that she, and women like her, are abusers because only a paedophile could see the potential for abuse in a situation where safeguarding has been compromised.

This doesn't make any sense when you calmly reflect on it. However, in the febrile context of social media, hundreds of transactivist accounts are promoting this narrative together, using highly emotive language to feign victimhood. Meanwhile, the mainstream press repeats these false accusations as if they have merit. The result is damage to the reputation of women and a vast amount of emotional labour being spent on appeasing highly distressed transactivists. Before you know it, everyone would rather the whole issue goes away, and for this, women need to shut up and stop provoking abuse.

It is not accidental that feminists are transactivists' biggest opponents. The bulk of feminist activism involves protecting women and children from male abusers, which usually consists of resisting some form of DARVO. Many feminists have also experienced DARVO in their private lives, if not from abusive partners, then from Men's Rights Activists who have been trying to roll back women's rights since their inception.

When feminists see a man campaigning to force girls to toilet, shower, and sleep next to genitally intact adult males, and he refers to women and girls who object to this as "bigots" and "child molesters," we recognise the pattern. We know that many people in our institutions recognise this pattern also, or they should do if they understand how safeguarding works and why it exists in the first place - not because all men are abusers but because abusers are so effective in manipulating others. Firm boundaries must always be in place to protect the vulnerable and help expose those who escalate when they come across a boundary they cannot easily transgress.

By using DARVO to engineer a climate of "no debate", trans-activists have successfully sidelined women's groups and presented themselves as the sole stakeholders in decisions that concern women's and children's rights. The outcome is the effective dismantling of child safeguarding, institutional policies that force women into dangerous situations in order to appease abusive men, and institutional paralysis around this issue.

However, as long as our institutions continue to justify their inaction, they will be enabling the abusers. The mask has well and truly slipped now. It is time for those in charge to find the courage to act.

Chapter 14

Our Society Can't Function If It Can't Tell the Difference Between Fantasy and Reality

It has become common for those who attempt to mediate a so-called "culture war" between transactivists and gender critical feminists to say that "both sides" need to stop behaving badly, even though there is no evidence of gender-critical women ever being violent toward transactivists or trans people. On the other hand, transactivists have staged masked protests and even threatened to bomb venues where women were meeting to discuss their rights. They have assaulted feminists and regularly misrepresented their position in order to discredit them. They also regularly intimidate women with death and rape threats.

Therefore, it is only the transactivists who have demonstrated an inability to engage with alternative points of view without resorting to abuse and violence. The evident fact that these attackers are consistently male, while their targets are female, should give anyone pause.

Physical vs metaphysical

The crux of the transactivist claim that "transwomen are women" is that "man" and "woman" are psychological or even "socially constructed", rather than biological, categories. According to them, a man is a woman if he says that he feels like a woman on the inside.

This is an argument rooted in metaphysics - a branch of philosophy that uses thought experiments to answer elusive questions such as what is being, knowing and identity. Thought experiments are highly subjective and prone to bias so metaphysical theories have no empirical proof, even though concepts such as self-awareness and identity have manifestations and consequences in the real world.

On the other hand, feminists maintain that men (adult human males) and women (adult human females) are two biological sexes that are necessary for our species to reproduce. Biological sex is *binary* in that there are only males and females. It is *determined at conception* when the sperm - which carries either an X or a Y chromosome - fertilises the egg - that always carries an X - to create a new life. From this moment onwards *every cell in our body* contains the same sex chromosome complement. If the cells have the Y chromosome, then the person is male. If the cells contain only X chromosomes, then the person is female.

To truly change our sex, the sex chromosome complement in our cells would need to be changed. Moreover, all the developmental processes and experiences of growing up as one sex would need to be undone and replaced with those of the opposite sex. Even if this was scientifically possible - and it isn't - the result would be a completely different person. This means that biological sex is *immutable*.

Biological sex in humans can easily be observed by just

looking at us, and this is especially true following puberty, when we acquire secondary sexual characteristics that amplify the underlying differences in size, muscle mass, proportions and reproductive roles. In rare cases of developmental ambiguities, our sex can still be determined by examining our sex chromosomes (karyotyping). All these claims are supported by empirical evidence.

Unfortunately, empirical evidence is not enough to settle the dispute between feminists and transactivists. Mainly because the societal belief in "psychological sex", "pink vs. blue brains", and the innateness of gender stereotypes of masculinity and femininity persists despite lack of evidence.

Ongoing brain scan research, which has been looking for empirical evidence to answer metaphysical questions such as where do identity and consciousness come from, has long been co-opted to give legitimacy to sexist prejudices. Previously, such studies were used to "prove" there is a neurobiological basis for women being nurturing, and good at housework, and for men being natural leaders and good at science. Today the same kind of studies are used to "prove" that people who identify as the opposite sex have "opposite sex brains".

So far, neuroscience has offered no conclusive proof in this area. Still, the allure of proving that the sexist stereotypes of femininity and masculinity are innate and that gender non-conformity is a psychological manifestation of being "born in the wrong body", is too strong for society and for the scientific community alike to allow them to dismiss transactivists claims as pseudoscientific nonsense.

The conflict of rights

For over a century, feminists have campaigned for women's rights because women's participation in public life, and their ability to escape abuse, were identified as the most urgent human rights issues women and children were facing.

The anti-feminist backlash was carried out in the physical – by utilising patriarchal systems and male violence – but it was justified with metaphysical theories about women's psyche and the innateness of gender stereotypes (OHCHR, 2014).

In order to mitigate the catastrophic effects of male supremacy on women's lives, women built and staffed women-only facilities - such as rape and domestic violence shelters, toilets and hospitals - and they kept rebuilding when these were damaged by angry men. Eventually, society reluctantly accepted that women had agency, human rights and the same inherent quality and potential as men, but the temptations of old beliefs remain. Male supremacy continues to thrive and men, as a class, are just as violent and antagonistic towards women's rights, today, as they were a hundred years ago. However, their access to female victims has been thwarted thanks to the existence of women-only spaces and services. Disappear these by making them mixed-sex, as transactivists are demanding when they claim that "transwomen are women", and women are back where they started - having to self-exclude from public life and essential services such as healthcare, sport and education, or accept the constant risk of male violence.

There are two institutions that women most rely on to safeguard them when they are vulnerable to male violence - the criminal justice system and medicine.

For years now, the police and the courts have been allowing male perpetrators, including rapists and murderers, to self-identify as women. This has resulted in male crimes being recorded as crimes committed by women, and some violent male perpetrators being housed in female prisons, where they have intimidated, harassed and even raped women.

Medicine has historically treated the male body as the default and neglected research on women, which has negatively affected female patients. In healthcare settings, women are also vulnerable to sexual assault and other forms of abuse by men. One would think that in the 21st century, medicine would want to address these issues in a way that would help women.

Instead, elite medical leadership has chosen to meet the demands of transactivists by making the word "woman" a taboo, unless it refers to males who self-identify as women. Meanwhile, women are dehumanised as "cervix havers", "menstruators", "chest feeders", "pregnant people" and even "bodies with vaginas" - a sexualised and dehumanising term which has found its way to the cover of The Lancet magazine (Bhvishya & Bunyan, 2021)

This kind of terminology is cynically referred to as "gender neutral language" and it is being deployed under the guise of "inclusivity". Women are told that both women who identify as men, as well as men who identify as women (or non-binary), don't like to be reminded of their biological sex, but that they too might want or need to use women-only services. Therefore "for the sake of clarity" the words "woman" and "female" are replaced with anatomical and physiological terms that are supposed to specify what type of body the service refers to.

Interestingly, the word "man" has entirely escaped this fate. You will not find any healthcare materials that refer to men as "prostate havers", "ejaculators" or "impregnators". More broadly, it is almost exclusively women-only facilities - hospital wards, lavatories and other single-sex spaces and services - that are being changed into "gender neutral" or "unisex".

In a blog titled "What it's like to be a transgender patient and a GP", which was published by the British Journal of General Practice, a trans-identifying male doctor wrote: "A lot of my patients were quite conservative — many female patients wore long clothes, or the hijab — but they allowed me to examine them despite my change. In fact, after my transition, they even allowed me to perform more intimate examinations that they did not let me do when I was a male GP." (Kamaruddin, 2017)

With one in five women reporting to have been sexually assaulted by a man, and sexual assaults, harassment and voyeurism mostly occurring in mixed-sex environments (Giligan, 2018), it is hardly surprising that most women request female-only providers for intimate examinations. One might think that a male doctor claiming to be a female would be a good case study to examine the conflict at hand; between women's rights to same-sex healthcare providers and trans-identifying people's demand to be validated as the opposite sex. Instead, the UK medical establishment sent a clear message to female patients by giving this trans-identifying male GP the 'Member of the Year RCGP Inspire Award', in 2019, without challenging his narrative in any way.

Workplaces haven't been spared this trend either. Under current self-identification practices, men - even those who look male, haven't transitioned in any way and who have built their lives, careers and salaries on male privilege - need only to state that they have a "female gender identity" for their employers to claim that they have employed a woman.

Transactivists claim that no man would go through the "ordeal" of falsely claiming to identify as a woman, but is saying "I'm a woman" in a society where everyone is treated as a hateful bigot unless they unquestioningly honour that statement really that difficult? Is it harder for employers to turn a blind eye to the risks of males identifying as women than overcoming the deeply ingrained prejudice against women? More challenging than dealing with the consequences of injuries to the male ego and navigating the minefield of sexual harassment, assault, and bullying in the workplace? It seems that gender self-identification is doing little more than enabling employers to develop increasingly elaborate ways to obscure the ongoing sex-based discrimination of women (such as low representation, the wage gap, family-unfriendly work practices, and the glass ceiling).

Mainstream women's rights groups haven't managed to resist the gender self-identification trend either. In 2013 a group called 50:50 Parliament was launched by Frances Scott, alongside a petition asking for equal representation of the sexes in UK politics. In 2016, they launched 'Ask Her To Stand' initiative which was meant to "inspire, encourage and support women on their way to Westminster". In 2018, at the #AskHerToStand event, the panel of women were asked whether they would be happy if half of Parliament were transwomen. Sal Brinton, former Liberal Democrat MP and a member of the House of Lords, said: "Absolutely. Transwomen are women and we support them." Instead of a challenge, she received cheers from the audience. (About 50:50, no date; Halpenny, 2018)

If the history of women's oppression is any indication, this worrying trend could eventually result in only men, and men who self-identify as women, being employed in decision-making positions. If this happens, the representation of women will once again be entirely in male hands.

The abuses committed by men against women during the time when women lacked political representation, and protected single-sex spaces, included marital rape, paedophilic marriages, extreme domestic violence, child abuse, poverty, slavery, murder and genocides such as witch huntings, honour killings, infant femicide and sex-selective abortions. It was only because of women organising, resisting male violence and speaking out about the horrors they endured at the whims of men, that men as a class could no longer justify turning a blind eye to this. Yet, they did turn a blind eye for as long as they could, and now they are doing it again under the guise of transactivism.

If women's sex-based rights are transphobia, then trans rights are misogyny

Anyone who looks beyond sloganeering about "trans rights" will find that the controversy and heated debate in fact revolve around the transactivist demand for the removal of women's sex-based rights, and women's objections to that.

Should transactivists stop fighting for gender self-identification tomorrow, trans people in the UK would still have the same rights as everyone else and they would continue to be one of the demographics least likely to be seriously harmed in our society (FPFW, 2017). Women, however, have much more to lose. If gender self-identification becomes legal tomorrow, women would not only continue to suffer endemic violence at the hands of men, they would have no safe places left to escape to.

Statistics world-wide show that men are responsible for the vast majority of violent crimes. According to the UK Ministry of Justice figures for 2019, men constituted 98% of those prosecuted of sex offences, 93% of those convicted of carrying weapons and 84% of those convicted of violence against the person. These figures are possibly even higher if we consider that the authorities have been recording violent crimes committed by men, who declare an opposite sex gender identity, as crimes committed by women. Meanwhile, women are far more likely to be victims of crime, with histories of abuse and violence toward them. (Her Majesty's Inspectorate of Probation, 2021)

We already know that gender-reassigned males retain male-pattern criminality (Dhejne, et al., 2011). We also know that transvestic fetishism tends to co-occur with other paraphilias (Abel, et al., 1988) and that over 50% of transgender inmates in UK prisons are sex offenders, compared to less than 20% in the ordinary male prison population (FPFW, 2017). So what possible justification could there be for allowing the practice of men self-identifying as women to continue?

When asked to comment on women's concerns that gender self-identification would increase male violence against women, Sophie-Grace Chappell, a trans-identified male philosopher and an "expert on GRA reform", said:

"Let me rightly dismiss that as scaremongering and would say, no look, it doesn't matter...It wouldn't matter actually if there was a slight spike in those statistics because this isn't about that kind of issue. It is about human rights. The fundamental thing is human rights and if we have problems resulting from that than we can address them." (Boyle, 2021)

When transactivists are asked about the human rights of women to not be assaulted by men accessing women's safe spaces, they tell us women's lives are acceptable collateral damage in order to "prevent trans people from killing themselves". The fact that these suicide-mongering claims have been debunked time and time again, doesn't seem to matter. This emotionally manipulative narrative has been incredibly successful in coercing society to go along with transactivist demands anyway.

None of this is to say that gender non-conforming people don't suffer discrimination in society - they do and have done historically. Homophobic bullying, in particular, can take an enormous toll on the quality of life and mental health of a person, as well as contribute to the development of opposite sex gender identity (DeLay, et al., 2017). With that in mind, let's examine whether gender self-identification is actually helpful or harmful to the demographic it purports to protect.

Limitations of gender self-identification

Only a minority of trans-identifying people pass as the opposite sex. This is not because people are "transphobic" or "uneducated" but because, beyond the law forcing people to pretend, we have an instinctive ability to correctly sex people regardless of mannerisms, clothes, makeup, surgery or politically correct instruction. This innate skill is essential for obvious reasons, such as relationships and risk assessment.

Furthermore, many trans-identifying people eventually stop taking cross-sex hormones - some due to the debilitating side effects and others because they realise that altering their bodies isn't a magical cure for dysphoria. Whenever this happens the body starts to revert to its original form although some interventions, such as the removal of breasts and genitals, are irreversible.

Gender-reassigned patients with dementia are also known to become very distressed when they realise parts of their anatomy are missing, or that they are wearing a dress and being addressed as if they were women, when they know themselves to be biologically male (BBC, 2018). This casts serious doubt on claims that opposite sex gender identity is in any way "inherent".

Despite this, trans-identifying adults and children are led to believe that transitioning is an act of "becoming their true selves", a one-way street at the end of which lies happiness and social acceptance. Transition regret, along with the reality of what these interventions can and cannot achieve - both medically and socially - are seldom discussed. Neither is the possibility of desistance. In fact, trans-identifying people who have experienced transition-related problems report that they have found themselves ejected from LGBT+ communities, and unable to access medical and psychological support, because their personal experiences provide an inconvenient challenge to the dominant transition narratives.

In the end, both women and transgender people are shortchanged by transactivism. The true beneficiary is the patriarchy, which includes the medical-industrial complex, which is profiteering from a growing gender reassignment industry.

The clash between transactivists and gender-critical women is just another clash between patriarchy and female liberation - as well as the clash between fantasy and reality, and between metaphysical and physical. In that clash, it is only the gender-critical perspective that is offering a robust intellectual analysis of our society and the power relations within it, while continuing to safeguard the vulnerable regardless of their age, sex or gender (all without threatening, attacking or censoring anyone).

Institutional failure

Widespread and uncritical pandering to the demands of transactivists is the result of a test that all our institutions have failed spectacularly, thanks to the incompetence of individuals and inadequacy of the safeguarding systems.

The test was simple, and answers were easily to be found in basic, mainstream science:

1. Humans are a sexually dimorphic species, whose sex is both determined at conception and immutable.

2. Women and girls are female while men and boys are male,

and this is true regardless of developmental abnormalities or self-declared identity.

3. Gender is a poorly defined concept with a meaning that ranges from socially constructed stereotypes and behaviour imposed on men and women, to being a euphemism for biological sex.

4. No law should be based on poorly defined and ambiguous terminology.

5. Male violence toward women is an endemic problem in our society.

For all these reasons, sex, not gender, is a protected characteristic under the Equality Act 2010, and institutions were supposed to uphold the protections enshrined in that law.

Universities were supposed to ensure that abstract theories weren't used to dismantle existing sex-based rights and protections. Instead, as postmodernism and queer theory came to dominate academia, we have witnessed an escalation of violence against women on campus. Female academics who tried to discuss how gender self-identification impacts women, such as Professors Selina Todd, Jo Phoenix, and Kathleen Stock, have been persecuted by students and staff. The list doesn't end there; you will struggle to find a woman who has tried speaking at a university about women's biology or sex-based rights in the last five years and hasn't been attacked, threatened, or even punished. From Lisa Keogh, Raquel Rosario Sanchez, and Julie Bindel to the Cambridge Radical Feminist Network and other women's groups, women at universities have been stymied in their attempts to speak about the biological reality of being a female or women's right to organise away from males.

The testimonies from university students and staff, which can be found on *gcacademianetwork.org* (GC Academia Network, no date) and in the Academia and Education section of the Institutional Capture page on my website (lascapigliata.com, 2021), are nothing short of shocking. Students and teachers alike speak of feeling afraid, self-censoring, and struggling to stand up for their beleaguered colleagues out of fear that they will become the next target. Their attackers justify their actions by offering new definitions of common words, such as "woman", "female," and "lesbian," and they deem anyone who refuses to follow the new orthodoxy as deserving of violence.

Gaslighting always starts in language, and travesties of the early 21st century illustrate this. Humanitarian wars (neo-colonialism), neoliberalism (techno-feudalism), collateral damage (war crimes), affirmative treatment (sterilisation of vulnerable minors), cotton ceiling (rape culture), sex work and pornography (sexual exploitation) all rely on the misuse of language to obscure abusive practices.

Therefore, upholding the meanings of words and adhering to observable reality is the only way to safeguard society against charismatic demagogues who rely on obfuscatory language and the weaponisation of symbols - as well as human hopes and fears - to bring about destruction.

Universities have always been places where fierce debates have thrived. They are also places where impressionable young minds come to be educated. Failing to safeguard free speech, and turning universities into indoctrination camps for aggressive ideologies, is an unforgivable failure. If historical events such as the Cultural Revolution in China are anything to go by, it is also potentially dangerous.

Law enforcement was supposed to accurately record a perpetrator's sex, and the media was supposed to accurately report it. If the concept of hate crimes was to be introduced, misogyny - ie. dislike of, contempt for, or ingrained prejudice against women - should have been on that list alongside the clear definition of women as adult human females, because oppression of women is rooted in our female biology.

Instead, by colluding in the self-identification of male offenders, men are being sent to women's prisons and sexually and physically assaulting women there, while a Hate Crime Bill in Scotland offers more protection to a man wearing a dress on a stag night than they do to women (Garton, 2021).

Prisons have always been segregated by sex due to the high risk of male violence against women. Since the advent of gender self-identification, policies that allow male perpetrators with or without a gender recognition certificate to be transferred to the female estate have become the norm. However, what is truly unforgivable is the callous disregard for women's suffering under these conditions.

When a woman who one such man sexually assaulted brought a Judicial Review against the Ministry of Justice, the male judge acknowledged the conflict of rights but ruled that this abhorrent practice was "capable of being operated lawfully", despite the danger it posed to women. (FPFW, 2021)

Schools should teach biology, not pseudoscience, and protect children from political lobby groups that promote medical and social interventions that harm gender non-conforming minors. They are also legally required to provide single-sex facilities to children over the age of 8.

Instead, girls' toilets have all but disappeared while the sexual assaults of girls (by boys) are increasing, and girls are starting to miss school during menstruation. Good initiatives such as sex and relationship education are being used to indoctrinate children into believing that if they have gender-atypical interests they could really be the opposite sex, while teachers are "socially transitioning" gender non-conforming minors and putting them in touch with lobby groups that advocate medical gender reassignment, all without informing their parents. (Braverman, 2022)

Medicine was supposed to adhere to the principles of evidence-based medicine. Instead, they allowed transactivism to influence medical treatment. Now, you will struggle to find a single medical or nursing body willing to discuss their close relationship with gender ideology lobby groups, the dangers of medical gender reassignment, or how gender self-identification harms female patients.

According to the NHS Pledge (Department of Health and Social Care, 2021) and CQC Guidance (CQC, 2015), the NHS was supposed to provide single-sex hospital accommodation. Instead, they have hidden from the public that men who self-identify as women have been admitted on women-only wards since at least 2010 (Harper-Write, 2018). All this has occurred despite male on female sexual violence, in a medical setting, being a serious and enduring issue.

Sporting bodies were supposed to safeguard both female athletes and female sport. Instead, they changed the rules without any scientific backing to allow male athletes to self identify into competing "as women". These males had the benefit of male puberty - which is irreversible. However, the sporting bodies allowed them to compete with elite women if they reduced testosterone, an intervention that is proven not to remove male sporting advantage (Hilton, et al., 2020). These male athletes now routinely take titles, records, awards and sponsorships from women and girls, while physically endangering them in team and contact sports. Disconcertingly, these male athletes are also reported to be exposing their genitals in the female locker rooms, while the concerns of the female athletes are being dismissed and ignored (Cohen, 2022).

Female-only shelters and rape crisis services

were created to provide single-sex services to vulnerable women and children. Instead they alienate women who are rape survivors, particularly those with PTSD, by forcing them to share accommodation with sexually inappropriate men who self identify as women (Brean, 2018; Shaw, 2019; Pazzano, 2014).

De facto gender self-identification has already resulted in biological males who self-identify as women entering rape crisis services as both service providers and service users (Finlay, 2021; ERCC, no date).

When asked to comment on female rape survivor's concerns about the disappearance of single-sex rape crisis services, a trans-identifying man who is employed as a chief executive of Rape Crisis Scotland alleged that such women are "bigoted" and that in his opinion they can't recover unless they "reframe their trauma" (FWS, 2021). At an event in Sheffield, he further alleged that Edinburgh Rape Crisis Centre - which is a service built by women, for women, to be a safe space to heal from male violence - "has been a trans inclusive space for a really long time.. so it had to really wash and clean its history of the perception of rape crisis centres not being inclusive of trans people." He acknowledged that women were self-excluding from this service due to the presence of men, but he followed it up by saying "we have to learn to be not transphobic, because our society is transphobic" and by smearing women who campaign for single-sex services as "being on the right and being very comfortable associating with fascists." (Hatchet, 2021)

LGBT+ organisations were supposed to advocate on behalf of lesbians, whose sexuality is a single-sex space. Instead, they have redefined same-sex attraction as "same-gender attraction", and they are branding lesbians "sexual racists" for refusing to have sex with men who identify as women (Bartosch, 2021).

They are also lobbying the government to remove single-sex exemptions from the Equality Act 2010 (WPUK, 2018).

By redefining "women" to include a subset of men, our institutions have given primacy to the poorly defined and metaphysical concept of "gender identity" over the material reality of inhabiting a female body. The same female body which is violated, oppressed and exploited by men in the real world. By doing this, they have destroyed any safe spaces - physically and metaphysically - where women could retreat to heal, be safe and organise away from men. More, even, than making men the default human being, they have made "women" a figment of men's imaginations. They have disembodied us as social beings. They have dehumanised and endangered us, I dare say, like never before.

Many trans-identifying people genuinely struggle with accepting their bodies and report temporary relief from "gender dysphoria" by presenting as the opposite sex. However, there is a difference between presenting as the opposite sex and the use of violence and the might of patriarchal institutions to compel society to pretend there is no material difference between being the opposite sex and feeling like the opposite sex.

People who suffer oppression for their bodies, such as ethnic minorities, women, and the disabled, don't have the luxury to identify out of it. Yet, our institutions continue to promote the belief that the most oppressed group in history consists of healthy and often privileged people - such as white middle class men - who are self-identifying into oppressed groups using the phrase "born in the wrong body". Thanks to not suffering the same limitations experienced by groups they wish to be part of, they exert immense influence on the regulators and these communities, where they position themselves as leaders and spokespeople. They are then redefining the aims and priorities of those groups and preventing genuine members from freely discussing issues that affect them.

Instead of considering the concerns of all the stakeholders in this conflict of rights, our institutions have complied with the transactivist assertion that any opposition to their ideology is a "transphobic". This has so far generated multiple, rather confused, inquiries, such as the inquiry into the proposed changes to the Gender Recognition Act, the inquiry into Disorders/Variations of Sex Development and, most recently, the inquiry into the proposed ban on Conversion Therapies. When the language, goals and aims are muddled by gender identity ideology, any attempts to address real-life discrimination and inequalities is sabotaged from the outset.

All levels of education, from kindergarten onwards, help equip us for life in the real world by teaching us the difference between fantasy and reality. Knowing how to prioritise the real over the imaginary helps us survive, because wishing for something doesn't automatically make it so. Some things can be changed, others cannot, and accepting the limits the real world imposes on our inner vision not only allows us to direct our energy and resources appropriately, it helps us to develop compassion toward others and ourselves, too. Thanks to the uncritical acceptance of transactivists' demands, we are at risk of losing this ability.

It's not accidental that sex is the subject of this institutional failure. Sex-based oppression of women by men is fundamental to how our society is organised, and our institutions were always a part of that. However, by allowing fantasy to trump reality on an increasing number of issues, the social contract is in danger of being broken. Even if it looks like this will benefit men as a class, it won't stay that way for long. In addition to women being disenfranchised, our whole society will suffer the consequences of giving primacy to feelings over facts. Climate change, environmental damage, vaccines and poverty are all burning issues that have been muddled by ideology. The longer we are unwilling to separate fact and opinion, reality and fantasy, truth and a lie, the more likely we are to lose the ability to function in the real world.

Bibliography

OHCHR. (2014). Gender stereotypes and Stereotyping and women's rights. United Nations Human Rights Office of the High Commissioner. https://www.ohchr.org/sites/default/files/Documents/Issues/Women/WRGS/OnePagers/Gender_stereotyping.pdf

Bhvishya, P. Bunyan, R. (2021). Lancet editor apologises for calling women 'bodies with vaginas' on medical journal's cover. Mail Online. https://www.dailymail.co.uk/news/article-10035415/Lancet-editor-apologises-calling-women-bodies-vaginas-medical-journals-cover.html

Kamaruddin, K. (2017). What it's like to be a transgender patient and a GP. British British Journal of General Practice 2017; 67 (660): 313. DOI: https://doi.org/10.3399/bjgp17X691433

Gilligan, A. (2018). Unisex changing rooms put women in dange. Our investigation shows single-sex facilities are far safer. The Times. https://www.thetimes.co.uk/article/unisex-changing-rooms-put-women-in-danger-8lwbp8kgk

About 50:50. https://5050parliament.co.uk/about/

Halpenny, C. (2018). When asked if the panel would be happy if half of Parliament were trans women, @SalBrinton says: "Absolutely. Trans women are women. And we support them." Cue subsequent cheers from the audience Raising hands Two hearts #AskHerToStand. https://mobile.twitter.com/ccchloe/status/1019633671853301762

FPFW. (2017). How often are transgender people murdered? https://fairplayforwomen.com/trans-murder-rates/

Her Majesty's Inspectorate of Probation, (2021). Specific sub-groups - Women. https://www.justiceinspectorates.gov.uk/hmiprobation/research/the-evidence-base-probation/specific-sub-groups/women/

Dhejne, C. Lichtenstein, P. Boman, M. Johansson, A. L. V. Långström, N. Landén, M. (2011). Long-Term Follow-Up of Transsexual Persons Undergoing Sex Reassignment Surgery: Cohort Study in Sweden. PLoS ONE 6(2): e16885. https://doi.org/10.1371/journal.pone.0016885

Abel, G. Becker, J. Cunningham-Rathner, J. Mittelman, M. Rouleau, J. (1988). Multiple Paraphilic Diagnoses among Sex Offenders. The Bulletin of the American Academy of Psychiatry and the Law, 16(2), 153–168.

https://www.researchgate.net/profile/Mary-Mittelman/publication/19760035_Multiple_paraphilic_diagnoses_among_sex_offenders/links/02bfe5109e71babeb3000000/Multiple-paraphilic-diagnoses-among-sex-offenders.pdf?origin=publication_detail

FPFW. (2017). Half of all transgender prisoners are sex offenders or dangerous category A inmates. Fair Play for Women. https://fairplayforwomen.com/transgender-prisoners/

Boyle, E. (2021). Nicola Sturgeon under fire after 'not valid' women's concerns comments. https://www.express.co.uk/news/politics/1494096/Nicola-sturgeon-news-first-minister-backlash-gender-recognition-act

DeLay, D. Lynn Martin, C. Cook, R. E. & Hanish, L. D. (2018). The Influence of Peers During Adolescence: Does Homophobic Name Calling by Peers Change Gender Identity?. Journal of youth and adolescence, 47(3), 636–649. https://doi.org/10.1007/s10964-017-0749-6. https://pubmed.ncbi.nlm.nih.gov/29032442/

BBC. (2018). Dementia care advice for transgender patients drawn up. https://www.bbc.co.uk/news/uk-wales-43365446

GC Academia Network. https://www.gcacademianetwork.org

lascapigliata.com (2021). Institutional capture testimonies. https://lascapigliata.com/institutional-capture/

Garton, A. (2021). BILL FURY: Hate Crime Bill: Humza Yousaf faces anger as law gives protection for 'cross-dressers' but not women. The Sun. https://www.thescottishsun.co.uk/news/politics/6803680/hate-crime-bill-scotland-free-speech/

FPFW. (2021). Transgender prison policy: judicial review ruling confirms trans rights do conflict with women's rights. Fair Play For Women. https://fairplayforwomen.com/transgender-prison-policy-judicial-review-ruling-confirms-trans-rights-do-conflict-with-womens-rights/

Braverman, S. (2022). Schools should know the law on trans rights. https://www.telegraph.co.uk/news/2022/08/09/schools-should-know-law-trans-rights/

Department of Health and Social Care (2021) The NHS Constitution for England. https://www.gov.uk/government/publications/the-nhs-constitution-for-england/the-nhs-constitution-for-england

CQC (2015) Guidance for providers on meeting the regulations, Care Quality Commission. https://www.cqc.org.uk/sites/default/files/20150324_guidance_providers_meeting_regulations_01.pdf

Harper-Write, A. (2018). Sex, Gender & the NHS. https://medium.com/@anneharperwright/sex-gender-the-nhs-1e8f4e6363a6

Hilton, E.N. Lundberg, T.R. Transgender Women in The Female Category of Sport: Is the Male Performance Advantage Removed by Testosterone Suppression?. Preprints 2020, 2020050226 (doi: 10.20944/preprints202005.0226.v1). https://www.preprints.org/manuscript/202005.0226/v1

Cohen, S. (2022). EXCLUSIVE: 'We're uncomfortable in our own locker room.' Lia Thomas' UPenn teammate tells how the trans swimmer doesn't always cover up her male genitals when changing and their concerns go ignored by their coach. Mail Online. https://www.dailymail.co.uk/news/article-10445679/Lia-Thomas-UPenn-teammate-says-trans-swimmer-doesnt-cover-genitals-locker-room.html

Brean, J. (2018). Forced to share a room with transgender woman in Toronto shelter, sex abuse victim files human rights complaint. National Post. https://nationalpost.com/news/canada/kristi-hanna-human-rights-complaint-transgender-woman-toronto-shelter

Shaw, D. (2019). Women's Refuge Opens Doors to Male, Transgender, Who Threatened to Kill Female Partner Continue reading Women's Refuge Opens Doors to Male, Transgender, Who Threatened to Kill Female Partner. Women Are Human. https://www.womenarehuman.com/womens-refuge-allows-male-transgender-who-threatened-to-kill-his-female-partner/

Pazzano, S. (2014). Predator who claimed to be transgender declared dangerous offender. Toronto Sun. https://torontosun.com/2014/02/26/predator-who-claimed-to-be-transgender-declared-dangerous-offender

Finley, K. (2021). Rape Crisis Centre Selects Male as CEO Despite Position Being Open to Women Only Continue reading Rape Crisis Centre Selects Male as CEO Despite Position Being Open to Women Only. Women Are Human. https://www.womenarehuman.com/rape-crisis-centre-selects-male-as-ceo-despite-position-being-open-to-women-only/

ERCC. (2022). Who we support and what are our services. Edinburgh Rape Crisis Centre. https://www.ercc.scot/who-we-support-and-our-services/

For Women Scotland. (2021). The real crisis at Rape Crisis Scotland. https://forwomen.scot/tag/mridul-wadhwa/

Hatchet, J. (2021). Unclean - Mridul Wadhwa wants to "clean" women out of Edinburgh Rape Crisis history. The Critic. https://thecritic.co.uk/unclean/

Bartosch, J. (2021). Trans lobby group Stonewall brands lesbians 'sexual racists' for raising concerns about being pressured into having sex with transgender women who still have male genitals. Mail Online. https://www.daily

mail.co.uk/news/article-10225111/Stonewall-brands-lesbians-sexual-racists-raising-concerns-sex-transgender-women.html

WPUK. (2018). Evidence of calls to remove single-sex exemptions from the Equality Act. https://womansplaceuk.org/2018/06/25/references-to-removal-of-single-sex-exemptions/

Chapter 15

On Symbols and Totalitarianism

Symbols are so integral to human thought and communication that man has been described as "symbol-using, symbol making, and symbol misusing animal" (Burke, 1966). Carl Jung, however, makes a distinction between *symbols* - which can mean different things to different people, as well as communicate concepts that are difficult to articulate, and *signs* - which are agreed by social convention to have a concrete and unambiguous meaning, such as letters of the alphabet, a stop sign or insignia on a uniform that identifies the wearer. He explained that "the sign is always less than the concept it represents, while a symbol always stands for something more than its obvious and immediate meaning. Symbols, moreover, are natural and spontaneous products". (Jung, 1964).

One example of this is the rainbow.

Even before language, art, and the written word were developed, natural rainbows inspired similar feelings in our ancestors as they do in us today - gentle rain bathed in sunlight feels like a promise of better things to come. Over the centuries, many ideologies and individuals drew rainbows to represent peace, hope, and benevolent higher power.

Then, in the late 1970s, the US gay rights activist Clive Baker turned the rainbow symbol into a rainbow flag.

Baker famously stated that flags were about proclaiming power, and the rainbow flag certainly delivered on this promise. Under its banner, the LGB (lesbian, gay and bisexual) community went from the "love that dare not speak its name" to a political movement that reclaimed their human right to a life free from discrimination and violence. These successes energised the rainbow flag further, giving it more power and greater social currency.

Then, the rainbow flag was misappropriated by trans rights activists.

"There is no LGB without the T, because LGBs owe their rights to trans women," trans rights activists said as they overlaid the pink, white and blue colours over the rainbow flag, to signify the enforcement of feminine and masculine gender stereotypes, which are to become a part of LGBT activism. "Did you know it was Marsha P Johnson - a trans woman - who threw the first brick during Stonewall riots?"

Marsha P. Johnson, aka Malcolm Michaels Jr., was a gay man and a drag queen who denied being present when the Stonewall riots started. In fact it was Stormé DeLarverie, a butch lesbian who fought the police as they tried to arrest her, that sparked the Stonewall riots by asking the onlookers "Why don't you guys do something?!". When the policeman threw her into the back of the police van, the crowd went "berserk" and the rest is history.

"Since the LGBs owe their rights to the T," transactivists press on, ignoring the facts, "T should be centred in LGBT activism. By the way, it's LGBTQ now because all "queers" belong under the rainbow flag too. What, you object to the term "queer" because it was used as a slur against LGB people? Don't worry. We have reclaimed the slur on your behalf. "Queer" is a lot more inclusive - people with kinks and fetishes, as well as heterosexual people with blue hair, are all "queer" now. We added a + at the end of the acronym to include sex workers, intersex people, and anyone else who might want to be involved in our activism. Let's overlay more colours and symbols over the rainbow flag to represent them all!"

When gender identity was force-teamed with sexual orientation, the rainbow flag really took off as a symbol of power. Today, it is hard to spend an hour online without encountering the familiar sequence of colourful stripes. Professional logos are changed to incorporate it. Police cars are covered in it. Town Halls are flying it. Zebra crossings are painted with it - despite authorities being aware that police horses, as well as people with sensory processing difficulties, are disturbed by its bright colours.

Of course, there is Pride, too - Pride march, Pride parade, Pride week, Pride month - all of which are designed to celebrate anyone who claims the rainbow - now known as the Pride flag. Even when they shout "Die cis scum!", burn effigies of lesbian feminists and celebrate rubber fetishism, adult babies and BDSM at ostensibly "family friendly" Pride marches, the magical sequence of the colour spectrum instantly transforms bad, anti-social and threatening behaviours into inherently brave, righteous and virtuous activism.

Whenever I have criticised totalitarian forces who have draped themselves in rainbow flags, I've encountered a knee jerk response from people who, although agreeing that this symbol has been misused, still maintain that the rainbow flag should be above criticism because of its origins. I understand this sentiment. The rainbow flag has been an important political symbol and a force for good for over half a century. However, having witnessed human rights abuses and bloodshed being carried out in the name of flags, my alarm bells go off whenever I am told that symbols must not be questioned.

* * *

I will never forget the summer of 1990. I was spending my summer holidays in my grandparents house on the Croatian coast, like every summer before that. The weather was beautiful and the sea warm and sparkling blue. The atmosphere, however, was palpably different. The civil war was brewing between Serbs and Croats, and there was fear in the air; the fear of a fragile peace between two nations ending, and what horrors that would bring.

During WWII, the Independent State of Croatia exterminated hundreds of thousands of Serbs in a genocidal campaign of ethnic cleansing. The Yugoslavia I knew and loved was riddled with monuments that had been erected on the sites of former concentration camps and mass graves. This is why, while Serbs may have agreed to live with the Croats in the same country after the war, this peaceful co-existence was conditional on numerous failsafe mechanisms being implemented, including a ban on symbols of Croatian nationalism.

In their bid for independence from Yugoslavia, and in defiance of the rules they felt were stifling, Croatian political leadership raised a flag that was nearly identical to the red, white and blue one featuring a red and white checkerboard coat of arms, under which so many Serbs had perished before. If this was designed to radicalise Croats and provoke the Serbs, it certainly worked. By the following year, the Serbs, who were some 15% of the total population of Croatia and a majority in some areas of so-called "Serbian Krajina", were being fired from their jobs, they were talked about in the media using dehumanising language, many were physically threatened and some were even taken from their homes and murdered (Wikipedia, no date).

It didn't take long for the Serbs in Krajina to respond by declaring their autonomy and allegiance to Yugoslavia. They dug up the WWII weapons they had hidden in their stables for just such an occasion, barricaded the roads and rejected Croatian independence. They also raised a flag - the red, blue and white flag of the Serbian republic, only instead of a socialist red star, it sported a white cross and four fire steels, to symbolise the Serbian Orthodox church.

As the violent clashes escalated, Croatia unilaterally declared independence and pronounced Serbs the enemies of the state. Civil war ensued, I'm sure you've heard about it.

During this war, the Serbian population in Croatia was reduced once again, as ordinary citizens were exiled and murdered in the name of the flag, which to many symbolised the past glory of the Independent State of Croatia and its power over its neighbours. The flag is venerated by many Croatians, to this day, with no remorse for the vast human tragedy that was perpetrated in its name. Serbs still loathe it, and perhaps always will. To stop hating that flag would mean the betrayal of all those who suffered under it.

I am sure Croatians have similar feelings about the Serbian flag - although for different reasons - and more widely, all Balkan tribes have their own stories to tell about the symbols they fear and despise, and the bloody feuds that define much of our history.

It's difficult to know what the future holds for the beleaguered Balkans, especially considering turbulent politics, shifting allegiances and the fact we've been stuck together since antiquity, doomed to be pawns in the power struggles between big players on the world stage. The raising of the two flags certainly symbolised the end of an era. A momentous change that is felt but not fully understood.

* * *

What's stayed with me after all these years is a feeling of unease with the way symbols are used to create insignia, which are then revered and elevated above criticism.

Totalitarian regimes often masquerade as "progressive" in the beginning. They profess love, unity and protection and they use well-loved symbols to convince passionate yet gullible people, who may not be familiar with the history or have the life experience to spot warning signs, to act as ideological foot soldiers. This is how we got to a point where the official LGBT+ organisations are maligning and attacking gay men and lesbians for being same-sex attracted. As they do this under the rainbow flag, and while repeating mantras about inclusivity and tolerance, anyone who points out their wrongdoing is automatically accused of bigotry and hate.

Social media driven cancel culture is the instrument of force here, and if you've been paying any attention to the harms that have occurred in the name of the rainbow flag - the sterilisation of gender non-conforming minors, the eradication of women's single sex spaces, male abusers gaining access to female prisons, shelters and bathrooms - you will know that we are knee deep in totalitarian chaos already.

I don't know how much destruction needs to happen before we are officially allowed to criticise what the rainbow flag has come to represent, but I can tell you this much: my life and the lives of my ancestors have been marked by the abuse of symbols and the humanitarian catastrophes that follow them. I don't care about false accusations, outraged gasps or side-eye glances when I talk about this. I will speak against totalitarianism wherever I see it.

If we care about our future, we must keep in mind that there are no sacred cows. There are just people and their suffering, and that needs to be your moral compass and your impetus, not a colourful piece of cloth, a name, or a symbol you can worship above all else.

Bibliography

Burke, K. (1966). Language as Symbolic Action. Berkeley & Los Angeles: University of California Press, p. 16

Jung, C.G., (1964), Man and His Symbols. Anchor Press. p.55

Wikipedia. Murder of the Zec family. https://en.wikipedia.org/wiki/Murder_of_the_Zec_family

Chapter 16

Letter to a Female Transactivist

I saw you in the crowd. You were holding up a placard covered in misogynistic slurs aimed at me. You and your male comrades shouted that I was a "TERF" and a "SWERF" - a trans-exclusionary and sex-worker exclusionary radical feminist - an accusation that sounded a lot like "feminazi", "witch", "bitch". Then you donned a balaclava, blocked the path of women who could be your mothers and grandmothers, and started to abuse and intimidate us. You had never met us before or heard what we had to say. You ignored the trans-identifying man who came out to ask you not to use him as an excuse to prevent our peaceful gathering. When he invited you to come in and debate with us, you refused. You said that "trans women" were "your sisters" and that you had no issue with them using women's toilets. When we told you some of us were rape survivors and that you don't have our consent to give away women-only spaces, you accused us of "weaponising our trauma".

There are 3.8 billion women on this planet, all of whom are

harmed in myriad ways by male violence and misogyny. We spent hundreds of years fighting for the rights and protections women and girls now have, and we are not going to allow a bunch of privileged university students, drunk on postmodernism, who have no life experience or understanding of the issues, to jeopardise our lives. We are not going to allow you to jeopardise *your* life. So listen up.

A man is not a woman. There's no medical procedure that can change sex in humans or any other mammal. When you fight for the right of men to call themselves "women" and to enter women-only spaces on the basis of their say so, you are doing what Men's Rights Activists have always done. You are violating women's boundaries for personal gain. You are allowing men to colonise women's spaces. You are creating a climate of fear which causes women and girls to withdraw from public life, because any semblance of safety – given by access to sex segregated spaces in situations where women are vulnerable – has been destroyed. Your activism is not feminism, it's at best misguided naivete, and at worst opportunism. By the time you realise how foolish you've been - because after all you are "just" a woman in your male comrades' eyes - it'll be too late.

The way entitled men disrespect women, the way they mow women down, the way they put their own needs, feelings and wants before women's lives and livelihoods, means they will do the same to you when you're no longer useful to them.

I'm sorry to say, but you are not original. History is full of women who thought they could bargain their way out of oppression by throwing other women under the bus. Women who believe that if only they joined in with the persecution of feminists, lesbians, women in prison and domestic violence shelters, they would be immune from attack. Believe this at your peril.

You might think it is "kind" and "progressive" to chant "trans women are women", but there are many things you don't yet know. Things you cannot know unless you are willing to listen to that group you malign now but will belong to soon enough - older women. Mothers. Mumsnet users. Women who understand on a visceral level - even if they don't want to, even if it's hard and inconvenient - the dangers inherent in prioritising male demands for validation over women's need for privacy, safety and dignity. You don't have to believe me, just reserve your judgement until you've had a few pap smears, a couple of kids, a full time job and a crappy marriage, perhaps a chronic illness or a sexual assault if you are unlucky, because then you'll be able to fully appreciate how the rights women have won don't actually translate to reality at the best of times, and how precarious they really are.

A woman I greatly admire, Penny White, once explained why it's so hard for young women to be feminists. You are young and whether you have a biological imperative to couple with men or not, you have no societal power. You are still very much in the throes of growing up, trying to figure out who you are, what you want to do with your life and where you belong. The patriarchy relies on convincing young women to ignore and despise older women. It's always worked hard on interrupting the flow of information between us, and this latest iteration of anti-feminist backlash is no different.

So, I get why it's not easy for you to put your head above the parapet. I was in your position once too, believe it or not. But now your understandable unwillingness to do the work of feminism has been weaponised against all of us.

I know you are not stupid and that there were times you felt something wasn't quite right about your comrades expecting you to pretend you were privileged compared to men who claim to be women. I also know that you have little choice but to maintain your cognitive dissonance or risk offending "liberal" men and being ostracised by your peers.

So you do what you're told. You campaign for men's right to masturbate to violent pornography and purchase sex from women who were trafficked and sexually abused as children. You enable these men to hurl misogynistic abuse at women because you do it alongside them, all the while celebrating them as some kind of rare unicorns, the "male feminists" who are so much better than those vile "man-spreaders" on public transport, or the "incels" you are allowed to denounce.

Are they better, though? Take the example of the transactivist art exhibited in 2018 at a San Francisco library. Nothing quite says "poor oppressed trans women" like a baseball bat wrapped in barbed wire, an axe covered in transgender flag colours, or a blood-stained shirt proclaiming, "I punch TERFs", does it?

Is there a higher, more noble feminist cause you could be fighting, than enabling male sex offenders to "identify as women" and enter women's hospital wards, prisons and DV shelters?

Have you thought about why, in the UK and Ireland, we can't stop men who identify as women from competing in women's sporting events, becoming Women's Officers and winning "Woman of the Year" awards, but women who identify as men still can't inherit peerages or become Catholic priests?

It's because this ideology you are caught up in is patriarchy on steroids, designed to rig the game even more to women's disadvantage.

You are probably thinking about your awkward male friend from uni, who looks a bit anxious in his blue lippy and a mini skirt, and you are about to say, "what a sweetheart, he wouldn't hurt a fly, only a monster would kick him out of women's spaces and groups". Please understand, to allow your friend to self-identify as a woman means you must respect any rapist or child killer when he does the same. Before you mention those "intense psychological assessments" that supposedly precede GRCs, remember that you are campaigning to remove them all. That's what gender self-identification means – any man can say he is a woman and automatically gain entry into women-only spaces. Even if for every hundred harmless "gender-bending" men you only get a couple of sexual predators who will take advantage of your activism to gain easier access to victims, how many women and girls are you prepared to sacrifice for your ideology? If in a bowl full of apples just one was laced with a lethal dose of cyanide, and there was no way of ascertaining which apple would kill you and which one is safe to eat, would you eat an apple from that bowl? I didn't think so.

Now for the good news: I think things are getting better.

Transctivism has highlighted the fact that as a society we aren't very well-versed in history, logic or critical thinking. Look at the climate change deniers, warmongers and anti-vaxxers everywhere, and how difficult it has become to convince people through reasonable arguments and scientific evidence. The adult world you are entering no doubt seems like a hot mess, where many species including our own are in existential peril. I'm sorry to put the weight of this on your shoulders, but you must do better. We all depend on you, like you will depend on your children one day, to undo your own mistakes.

I know that's a lot of pressure and a big ask, but every generation has its benefits and challenges. You can vote, go to University, divorce, run a business, have reproductive freedom and autonomy over your own body. Today rape is illegal in most places and you have profited from older women paving the way, through initiatives such as second wave feminism, #MeToo and #Time'sUp.

You see women in positions of power, even if they are rare. You can name a woman president, doctor, lawyer, teacher or Nobel Prize winner. Women older than you have won the right to protect children from abuse. We have dreamed of this for thousands of years, and you get to take it for granted.

These rights aren't unalienable. There's a reason why men didn't see fit to allow women equal rights for so long, and why women were put through medical and sexual torture, force-fed, starved, lobotomised, incarcerated, why they were even burnt at the stake as witches, before basic human rights were granted to them.

Something's gone wrong with men-kind. Whether it's nature or nurture, time will tell, but their fury and violence toward non-submissive women is a chronic epidemic that comes in waves. This is your wave. We need you to fight in our corner, not theirs.

There are loads of men who will accept you without forcing you to work against the rights of women and children - trust me on this. They'll also be much less entitled to your body, a lot less selfish, more mature and with a bit of luck, they won't even be porn-sick. They'll be better sharers, more honest and more accepting of their own flaws. Ok, this last one is probably my wishful thinking, as I haven't met a man yet who didn't have to be dragged screaming into an apology. Even so, if you raise your standards about male behaviour, you will only miss out on the jerks. You are much better off without those, no matter how cute they are.

The gender ideology you are being fed is a string of extraordinary claims that rely on groupthink and enforced compliance instead of being rooted in evidence. Being a woman is not a feeling. Women can't "identify" out of sex-based oppression any more than men can identify into it. This is why men's emotions and their need for validation should never be allowed to trump the right of women and children to be safe from male violence.

It was Lierre Keith who said, "Gender is not a binary, it is a hierarchy. Global in its reach, sadistic in its practice, murderous in its conclusion." Look her up and hear what she has to say. Then, when you are ready, come and join us.

Chapter 17

The Myth of Human Asexuality

In the sea of novel gender and sexual identities, one has become particularly prominent in recent years. It is called "asexuality," and it is often promoted in the media with photographs of young women dressed in sexy lingerie.

One such woman penned an article about the conflict between her "asexual identity" and the objectification she experienced as a young female model. How weird it felt to be instructed by photographers to flirt with the camera as if it was her boyfriend. How entering the modelling world made her worry that because of her body type, she would only ever be hired to shoot lingerie campaigns. How uncomfortable she was with the expectation to titillate and perform for the male gaze. How turning down a job that involved modelling BDSM gear led to her never getting the opportunity to work with that brand again.

She also told us that from a young age she had never had a particular interest in dating and relationships. This is not unusual. Most children find the idea of intimate relationships horrifying until they enter puberty and adolescence, and start maturing sexually. However, she claims to have never developed that interest, which is why she identifies as "asexual" (Benoit, 2019).

For a while now, women and girls have been adopting novel identities in order to signal their sexual boundaries to men. For example, in order to avoid being pressured into a one-night stand, a woman might say that she is "demisexual", which means that she only sleeps with, or feels sexually attracted to, those with whom she has formed a strong emotional bond or connection. If a guy still won't stop pestering her for sex, she just might resort to saying she is "asexual". Rather than rejecting him specifically, she is simply disinterested in sex altogether. No hard feelings.

Most women of any generation will recognise the creative ways in which women try to maintain sexual boundaries. Sex, after all, can be quite perilous for women, especially in the "hook up" culture that relies on online dating and meeting men without learning much, or anything at all, about them beforehand. Apart from pregnancy and STDs, we risk being coerced, raped and worse, especially since the escalation of violent pornography use among boys and men. However, instead of being acknowledged as boundaries, "demisexual", "asexual" and dozens of other made up words are being promoted as "identities".

You see, one is not a "frigid prude" or heaven forbid a "transphobic lesbian who won't have sex with penises". One is simply a "non-binary asexual", a "femme demi" or any other shiny new label that offers women escape from male sexual aggression, while giving them protection under the gender identity and sexual identity umbrella. Seeing LGBT+ charities promote "asexual identities" by giving them their own flag and a visibility week must seem reassuring for any woman or girl who wants to protect herself from unwanted sexual contact without risking being canceled and ostracised.

Reading about asexual identities in the LGBT+ press, however, you will quickly learn that many "asexuals" apparently have healthy libidos and masturbate just like anyone else. They just don't want to have sex with other people.

I can think of a few reasons beyond "identity" that could explain this.

Some people, and especially abuse survivors, might have healthy libidos but choose to steer clear of intimate relationships as a harm-avoidance strategy. Some men might favour intimate relationships with sex dolls or sex robots - for various reasons. Others prefer masturbation to sexual contact with another person due to narcissism, or psychosexual disorders such as "auto-eroticism" and autogynephilia - a condition where a man is sexually attracted to the idea of himself as a female sexual object, so he develops an erotic relationship with himself.

More worryingly, however, we are told that many "asexual" women love working as strippers and "sex workers" and that they "happily" submit to regular sexual activity - either with their husbands, boyfriends or clients - even though they neither enjoy sex nor want it.

Since I haven't found any stories of "asexual" men regularly making the same sacrifices for the benefit of their female partners, I am left with the overwhelming impression that rather than being a creative escape from sexual coercion, "asexual identities" smack of the same old patriarchal gaslighting that gave rise to the concepts of "wifely duties" and women being naturally "frigid", which have served to normalise the sexual exploitation of women, both in heterosexual relationships and in the context of porn, prostitution and wider rape culture.

It is not uncommon for women who claim to be "asexual" to

talk about the pressure to be sexy and flirty and having to feign sexual feelings in order to pander to the male gaze. I know a lot of women who can identify with that, and not because they are all "asexual".

Sex sells, and it is mostly women being paid by men to sell it with their bodies. Furthermore, a woman refusing to indulge an amorous man could agitate him, and an agitated man could lash out and hurt her, either physically, financially or professionally. So women flirt under duress, fake-laugh at men's innuendos and if a man won't stop pestering us for sex, we just might have to go along with whatever he wants, in the hope of quickly satisfying him so that he leaves us in peace. We listen to male sexologists claim that female orgasm is a myth, knowing that the real reason why so many women don't orgasm during penetrative sex is due to men being mainly interested in their own pleasure while sparing no thought for us as human beings with needs too. We roll our eyes at the conspicuous absence of the clitoris in anatomy atlases. We are horrified at the practice of a "husband stitch", where a doctor tightly sutures a vulva after labour, sacrificing a women's right to pain-free intercourse for the benefit of her husband's pleasure. We do this because despite fighting against male oppression for centuries, women still haven't found a way to make men stop abusing and exploiting us.

My hackles were further raised when I heard some doctors who work in paediatric gender reassignment cynically state that an absence of sexual desire and anorgasmia in young gender reassigned people might not be a side effect of puberty blockers and cross-sex hormones at all, but a sign that they were "always asexual".

It is well known that puberty blockers interfere with genital and sexual development, and patients of both sexes report an absence of libido and inability to orgasm in adolescence. This is further exacerbated by cross-sex hormones and genital surgeries such as penile inversion to create a "neo-vagina", which can be much more extensive and have a higher complication rate in patients with underdeveloped genitalia.

What's more, young people who are declaring "non-binary" and "asexual" identities are specifically targeted for so-called "nullification surgeries", which consist of removing genitals, breasts and even nipples altogether, so as to make one appear to be "sexless". This practice is a bizarre 21st century version of the Skoptsy cult, which did this to their followers to render them spiritually "pure" (Tulpe & Torchinov, 2000; Gluck, 2021).

While Skoptsy toured impoverished villages singing songs and promoting their religion, surgeons are now advertising "nullification" surgeries on platforms such as Instagram and TikTok, alongside young people who are proudly displaying their scars and missing anatomy. It doesn't stop there, though. The market for uterine implants for men is rearing its unethical head all the time, and guess where the young and healthy wombs are supposed to come from? If you thought they might come from the gender reassignment procedures, where young women are robbed of their reproductive organs in the name of "identities", you would be on the right track indeed.

Therefore, it is my concern that, in addition to sanitising transgression of women's boundaries, "asexual identity" might serve to obscure iatrogenic harm and ethical issues in the gender reassignment industry.

Quite apart from the current culture wars and modern ideologies, the idea of human "asexuality" doesn't make biological sense.

Humans are a sexually reproducing species, which means that males (who produce sperm) and females (who produce ova) need to have intercourse in order to create a new life. This process is facilitated by sexual attraction and sexual arousal, which are physiological functions, borne out of our anatomy and the biological imperative to procreate.

As human females don't outwardly signal ovulation, and both sexes are capable of experiencing sexual pleasure and orgasm, a lot of intercourse among humans occurs for bonding and pleasure purposes. So even though heterosexuality is the most common sexual orientation, homosexuality and bisexuality are well-recognised variants. These typically occur either in the context of experimentation during sexual maturation, or as lifelong sexual preferences in a proportion of individuals. There's even evidence that same-sex attraction expands the pool of caregivers, which makes it evolutionarily advantageous.

Therefore, even if a person has no desire or opportunity to pass on their genes, sexual attraction, arousal and bonding through intercourse and other forms of sexual intimacy are still a fundamental part of their biological make up.

Physiological urges motivate us to act, in order to relieve them. We eat to relieve hunger, sleep to relieve tiredness and have sex or masturbate to relieve sexual arousal. This urge-action-relief is a very basic mechanism by which even the simplest organisms, those which don't have complex brains, language or ability to think in abstract terms, can survive.

Like all fundamental urges, a sex drive has its rhythms, and there are ways in which it significantly differs from the lifelong daily imperative to satisfy sleep and hunger. Humans are born with a need to eat and sleep, but we don't develop a sex drive until puberty, and we don't need to act on it in order to stay alive. As our bodies mature sexually, however, our sex drive increases and remains high for some time, especially during early adulthood, when the chances of producing healthy offspring are the highest. Sex drive naturally decreases in later years, but even during fertile years, it waxes and wanes depending on hormonal cycles, lifestyle, environment, psychosocial stresses and the presence or absence of suitable mates.

While need-action-relief seems deceptively simple on the surface – I get hungry, I eat, I feel full, or I feel tired, I sleep, I wake up feeling rested - there is a whole host of behaviours and cultural practices that surround basic need fulfilment.

Hunger drives anything from food foraging, hunting, food preparation, farming, utensil making, kitchen design, recipe development and even division of labour within a home. Tiredness has compelled us to seek shelter in caves, skin animals to make comfortable lodgings, carve out four poster beds, sew wool into mattresses, develop cleansing routines, design silk pyjamas, and build houses with windows and locked doors, all so we can be safely unconscious for eight hours every night.

As children take a long time to gestate and even longer to mature and become independent, humans have developed many complex behaviours and rituals to manage the sexual urge too - from choosing a mate with the most compatible genes who is prepared to stick around and help us raise the young, to the long-term investment both parents make in producing offspring, which is reflected in our attitudes toward monogamy, marriage, divorce, division of labour and even ownership and property.

Not to mention the rituals involved in attracting the mate in the first place, which in humans involves a lot of deception, both thanks to beautification practices as well as not necessarily sincere promises of love and respect and to "treat you right".

Men fulfil their biological imperative to procreate by simply having sex and impregnating as many women as possible.

For women, this is only a start. Once they get pregnant, women have to grow the entire baby inside their bodies, give birth to it - which has a high risk of both infant and maternal mortality and morbidity - and then they have to feed the baby with their breast milk, care for it and continue raising and providing for all its basic needs for almost two decades, until the child becomes independent enough to live on their own.

Some men understand the role good husbands and fathers play in ensuring the health and well-being of the next generation, so they commit to the relationship and stick around in order to help the mother raise the child. Others do not, opting instead to walk out on their families.

I often wonder if this, in combination with the male strength advantage over women, has given rise to the gendered hierarchy and the systematic sexual coercion of females by males. In this system - which is known as patriarchy, male supremacy or the culture of male sexual entitlement - men have taken to treating women and children as possessions and resources, and relying on a game of numbers, rather than their own sacrifices and efforts, to ensure the survival of their offspring. Meanwhile, all the reproductive labour falls squarely on the shoulders of women, which further disadvantages them in this gendered hierarchy.

Be that as it may, by denying females their right to choose mates, normalising paternal abandonment and prioritising male pleasure and the male biological imperative over the needs of women and children, we have created a perfect storm around human sexuality.

Instead of sexuality being understood as a fundamental function our bodies are designed to fulfil – whether the goal is reproduction or not – and that sexual attraction to others serves a multitude of purposes, our culture has tabooed female sexuality, while organising itself around the exploitation of it. This has created an environment where sex and sexuality are never entirely free from the oppressive dynamics of the gender hierarchy - not the practice of it, not the research into it and not the safeguarding of the vulnerable from sexual abuse.

It should be said that, although low libido seems to be a more common phenomenon these days, the number of people who have *never* experienced sexual arousal or interest in sex is extremely low, and when it happens, the medical cause can usually be ascertained, regardless of whether treatment is available, or indeed desired, by the individual.

Some well-known medical and psychological conditions can cause a lack, or complete absence, of sex drive, as well as different kinds of sexual dysfunction. Side-effects of some widely prescribed medications, such as SSRIs, GnRH agonists or androgen antagonists, can cause low libido and anorgasmia. Erectile dysfunction in men has a whole host of causes, including cardiovascular illness, peripheral nerve damage due to diabetes, and overindulgence in masturbation as a part of porn addiction. Depression, anxiety, trauma, obsessive compulsive disorder and even some psychotic and personality disorders can cause a person to lose interest or to even be repulsed by the idea of having sex.

Celibacy - which has now been rebranded as an "asexual identity" - doesn't necessarily arise from these physical and psychological problems. It can be a lifestyle choice and one that's been celebrated in our society since antiquity. Not only as a behavioural strategy to minimise unwanted pregnancy, disease transmission and adultery, but men and women who declare the absence of sexual desire or vow not to relieve it through intercourse or masturbation, are seen as morally virtuous and spiritually pure.

As with so many other newly invented sexual and gender identities, "asexuality" is just a new word for several old concepts, dressed up in our current obsession with labelling ordinary things as something unique, stunning, and brave. These labels are a convenient distraction from the real work that needs to be done to address sexual exploitation and to teach everyone about healthy boundaries, bodily autonomy and the way our bodies work and why.

Instead of identities, we should focus on shedding some of the accumulated neuroses about sex and sexuality, and on working together to provide a safer space for all of us to exist as sexual beings.

Bibliography

Benoit, Y. (2019). I'm Asexual, And I'm A Lingerie Model. Here's How I Balance The Two. Huffington Post. https://www.huffingtonpost.co.uk/entry/asexual_uk_5d4bedfbe4b0066eb70d1f82

Tulpe, I. A. & Torchinov, E. A. (2000). The Castrati ("Skoptsy") sect in Russia: History, teaching, and religious practice. International Journal of Transpersonal Studies, 19(1), 77–87.. International Journal of Transpersonal Studies, 19 (1). http://dx.doi.org/10.24972/ijts.2000.19.1.77 https://digitalcommons.ciis.edu/cgi/viewcontent.cgi?article=1301&context=ijts-transpersonalstudies

Gluck, G. (2021). Castrating Children in the Service of Male Sexuality - Men's Fetishistic Practices Behind 'Gender Dysphoria'. https://genevievegluck.substack.com/p/castrating-children-in-the-service?r=dwf2a

Chapter 18

On Intersex, Transgender and Women's Sport

Humans are a sexually dimorphic species. This means that apart from reproductive and chromosomal differences, there are observable differences in appearance that account for why men are on average bigger, faster and stronger than women. Depending on the variable, there is more or less of an overlap between the sexes. Some women are taller and have more muscle than an average man and some men are shorter than an average woman, for example. However, these are the outliers. Overwhelmingly, men are able to dominate women due to superior strength, speed and aggression, and both endemic male violence against women and the fact that male athletes outperform female athletes in virtually every category, are stark reminders of this.

Due to the gendered power imbalance, sport has always been male-focused. Women's sport was created only recently, due to the advancement of women's rights and a recognition that without sex-segregated categories, there is little, if any, chance of fair play for women and girls.

It may therefore come as a surprise that today, males are allowed to compete in female sporting categories.

History of biological males in women's sport

From the outset, women's sport struggled to ensure female-only competition, mainly due to the inclusion of males who either masqueraded as women, underwent sex-reassignment surgery or had Disorders of Sex Development (DSDs).

As a result of these males outperforming women, in 1968, the International Olympic Committee sought to ensure fair play in women's sport by mandating on-site "sex checks" for female athletes. These initially consisted of visual observation and gynaecological exams, but this was quickly abandoned in favour of the much less traumatic genetic testing, which initially looked for X-chromatin (second, inactive X chromosome) as proof of female sex, and later on, the Y-chromosome as evidence of male sex.

This practice continued, not without controversy, until 1998 (Elsas, et al., 2000).

Because chromosomal sex checks could not differentiate between different DSD conditions - some of which gave 46 XY DSD males a female appearance and an insurmountable performance disadvantage compared to elite males - these tests were seen as imperfect and discriminatory. Therefore, following a prolonged campaign for the rights of DSD males to compete as women, chromosomal sex checks were abandoned in 1999, and replaced with testosterone suppression rules, which limited testosterone levels in female competition to below 10 nmol/L.

This, by far, exceeds the normal female serum testosterone range of 0.5 - 2.4 nmol/L (with female testosterone levels in excess of 6.9 nmol/L being indicative of a serious disease such as adrenal or ovarian tumours). However, it has allowed the inclusion of DSD male athletes as well as female athletes with medical conditions that raise their testosterone above normal female level, in women's sport.

By convention, both female athletes with raised testosterone, and DSD male athletes with testosterone level in the male range, were referred to as "females with hyperandrogenism". So when studies were published claiming that there was an overlap in serum testosterone between elite men and elite women, it was not clear whether this was a bona fide physiological overlap between the sexes or if it resulted from the female category being inherently mixed-sex.

Testosterone doping, and the fact it can suppress endogenous testosterone in males leading to low levels, could have also affected these results.

In 2014, Ferguson-Smith & Bavington published a paper arguing against the testosterone suppression rules.

The authors noted that the incidence of 46 XY DSDs is less than 1:20 000 in the general population, yet these conditions are present in 1:421 female athletes.

Most of these DSD athletes either had complete or partial androgen insensitivity.

In addition to 46 XY chromosomes, athletes with complete androgen insensitivity syndrome (CAIS) have high levels of circulating testosterone, to which their bodies are almost completely resistant so they were exempt from testosterone suppression rules. The athletes with partial androgen insensitivity (PAIS) however, had to undertake measures to lower their testosterone, either by having their testicles removed before entering competitive female sport, or by taking testosterone suppression drugs.

As a result of the sporting performance of CAIS and PAIS

athletes being found to be comparable, while their testosterone levels were very different, the authors argued that the performance advantage of 46 XY DSD athletes cannot be due to testosterone.

Looking at gender verification reports, they also noted that 46 XY DSD athletes, in general, were closer in stature to the average male, and that they had greater lean body mass than females.

Males who have two Y chromosomes - such as 47 XYY - are particularly tall. On the other hand, 46 XX DSD females who have masculinised appearance, still have female body habitus. Therefore, the tall stature found in 46 XY DSD athletes appears to be associated with genes on the Y chromosome, or the modulation of stature genes found on autosomes by the Y chromosome.

In their paper, Ferguson-Smith & Bavington acknowledged that the Y chromosome was not the only factor contributing to taller stature, and that sporting advantage was likely to be multifactorial.

However, the evident male/female sex-differences in athletic performance across almost all sports, and even in the pre-pubertal stages of child development (Marta, et al., 2012), suggest that no practical intervention could fully mitigate the sporting advantage conferred by the Y chromosome itself.

At this point, the logical conclusion should have been to abandon testosterone rules, return to genetic testing in order to ensure women's sport was female only, and create a third category where 46 XY DSD athletes could compete fairly and without being forced to suppress their testosterone.

Instead, the authors called for withdrawal of the "regulations on hyperandrogenism", but instead of arguing for the third category, they claimed that "tallness, whether determined by genes on the Y or any other chromosome, offers an example of an acceptable variable that contributes to athletic success in elite female athletes including those with 46,XY DSD" and that there was "no evidence" 46 XY DSD male athletes "possess any physical attribute relevant to athletic performance that is neither attainable nor present in 46,XX women" (Ferguson-Smith & Bavington, 2014).

In the wake of ongoing controversy, Indian sprinter Dutee Chand claimed that because there were no testosterone suppression rules in men's sport, that these rules in women's sport constituted sex-based discrimination. I don't know the details of Chand's medical history, but based on articles I could access, Chand appears to have a 46 XY DSD.

Chand won the sex discrimination case, and in 2015, the testosterone suppression rule for "females with hyperandrogenism" was overturned.

At the same time, the IOC ruled that normally sexed trans-identifying males could be included in women's competition too, as long as they professed to have a "female gender identity" and could demonstrate that their serum testosterone level has been below 10 nmol/L for at least 12 months prior to their first competition. (International Olympic Committee, 2015).

The following year, all three medalists at the Women's 800 metres competition in 2016 Olympics in Rio, were 46 XY DSD males.

Following the race, the three female competitors, who missed out on the medals, embraced in defeat and said, "We see each other week in, week out, so we know how each other feel".

Lynsey Sharp, who came sixth, broke into tears and said that, "It was difficult to compete against Caster Semenya and other hyperandrogenic athletes after the rule to suppress testosterone levels was overturned." She also complained that the athletes were effectively competing in "two separate races".

Many spectators empathised with the female athlete's predicament. However, the IAAF General Secretary Pierre Wiesse's dismissed their concerns by saying that Caster Semenya, was "a woman, but maybe not 100 per cent".

Although the details of athletes' medical history were not publicly known at the time, Caster Semenya appears to have been born with 5-ARD (5-alpha-reductase deficiency), which is a male DSD caused by an X-linked genetic mutation. Babies with 5-ARD have 46 XY chromosomes and testes, however, due to a genetic defect, their bodies don't produce enough steroid 5-alpha reductase 2 - an enzyme which drives the development of male genitalia before birth.

Consequently, male babies with 5-ARD are born with ambiguous genitals, a micropenis, hypospadias or even female-appearing genitals. They can sometimes be mistaken for girls, or deliberately raised as girls, but if they are allowed to develop normally and their testicles aren't removed in a "gender assigning" procedure, the surge in testosterone at puberty will result in masculinisation of the body and an associated sporting advantage over female competitors.

Following the debacle in Rio, studies found that a natural serum testosterone level did confer sporting advantage in certain women's events, after all, and in 2018 the rules were changed yet again.

The new testosterone limit for androgen-sensitive DSD male athletes was set at 5 nmol/L, whereas biologically female athletes, and DSD male athletes who were completely resistant to testosterone, were exempt.

Having dominated female athletic competitions whenever they were not required to suppress testosterone, double Olympic 800m champion Caster Semenya's sporting advantage was reduced with testosterone suppressing drugs, which also caused significant side effects. Therefore, Semenya issued a legal challenge, asking for the testosterone suppression rule to be removed.

In 2019, Court of Arbitration for Sport upheld testosterone suppression rules, stating that 46 XY 5-ARD athletes – such as Semenya – have "circulating testosterone at the level of the male 46 XY population and not at the level of the female 46 XX population. This gives 46 XY 5-ARD athletes a significant sporting advantage over 46 XX female athletes" (Mokgadi Caster Semenya v. International Association of Athletics Federation, 2018; Ingle, 2019).

Semenya appealed this decision at the Swiss Supreme Court in 2020 and lost. This meant that Semenya wasn't able to defend Olympic 800-metre title at the Tokyo Olympics in 2021, or compete at any top meets in distances from 400 meters to the mile, unless they agreed to lower their testosterone level through medication or surgery (Dunbar & Imray, 2020).

Semenya continues to pursue this case at the European Court of Human Rights.

Meanwhile, the IOC announced that normally sexed trans-identified males were allowed to compete in women's categories at the 2020 Tokyo Olympics, subject to 2015 rules that required them to profess a "female gender identity" and have evidence that their testosterone didn't exceed 10 nmol/L for 12 months.

It appeared that the transactivist strategy of conflating sex with gender - and DSD with transgender - had finally succeeded. If gender identity and femininity, rather than biological sex, determined whether an athlete was male or female (a concept that has already been validated through the inclusion of DSD males in women's sport), then privileges reserved for DSD males could arguably be extended to normally sexed males who identify as women.

Several high profile female athletes and coaches spoke out

against the escalating unfairness and compromised safety of female athletes under the new rules. Others remained silent for the fear of losing sponsorships and their place on the team.

Scientists such as Dr Emma Hilton reviewed the available evidence and confirmed that male sporting advantage is significant - ranging from 10-50% depending on the sport - and it cannot be removed by testosterone suppression, especially in the case of males who went through normal male puberty (Hilton & Lundberg, 2020).

None of this made much difference. Ever since 2016 when trans-identifying males were allowed to compete "as women", they've dominated female competitions, even if they only ever had mediocre success while competing with other men, and were much older and less fit than their female competitors. When these males were allowed to participate in contact sports, women suffered serious injuries such as broken bones (Ralph, 2017) and skull fractures (Presley, 2021).

For a while, things looked pretty grim for female athletes. Sporting authorities seemed swept up in narratives of "inclusion" and the "human right" of certain males to compete with women, while sports commentators around the world celebrated the records these males were setting in women's sport.

Eventually, USA Powerlifting and then World Rugby banned trans-identifying males from women's competition (World Rugby, 2021). For this, both organisations were vilified by transactivists, who maintained that "inclusiveness" was all important, while safety and fair play for women and girls was secondary. As a result, most other sporting associations have given in to transactivist demands.

This culture war reached fever pitch during the Tokyo Olympics, which saw several trans-identifying males compete in female categories, including a trans-identifying male athlete who was a part of New Zealand's weightlifting team. Even though this athlete didn't win a medal - and some commentators remarked on apparent lack of effort during this competition in comparison with their previous results - their qualifying meant that a female athlete was deprived of a once-in-a-lifetime opportunity to compete at the highest level (FPFW, 2021).

All over the world, spectators and athletes of both sexes were shocked at the disrespect both the New Zealand weightlifting team and the IOC showed for fair play and women's sport. However, both organisations doubled down on their questionable decisions. The trans-identifying male weightlifter from New Zealand was given a "Sportswoman of the Year" award by the University of Otago, while the IOC decided to abandon the testosterone suppression rule altogether.

Since then, the controversy has moved to the University of Pennsylvania swimming team, which has allowed a trans-identified male swimmer to compete against women, resulting in never before seen records (Lohn, 2022), accusations of indecent exposure in the female changing room (Lord, 2022) and ongoing protests by female athletes (Rushing, 2022).

If women athletes thought they had it bad under the new rules, wait until they see the new-new rules, which dispense with any pretence of caring about women's safety or fair play. Women's sport is now open to any man who claims he feels like a woman, and it is up to the individual sport to decide where the boundaries lie, in a febrile climate that is rife with cancel culture and spurious accusations of transphobia (International Olympic Committee, 2021).

The Platonic ideal

As far as I can tell, the rationale for inclusion of male athletes in women's sport has always been two-fold – unfavourable comparison to the Platonic ideal of a man, and compassion for their predicament.

Growing up, many DSD male athletes had either a female or an androgynous appearance. They are often raised as girls and their superior athletic performance in female competitions contributes to them being chosen for teams and sporting events.

Now imagine what it must be like to be raised believing you were female, perhaps even an athletics champion, only to discover that the reason you performed so well is because you are biologically male?

Not only does this cast a shadow on your sporting achievements, it changes the way you think about yourself and your future. As females we expect to become mothers and we are treated a certain way by society. Learning that we are in fact male not only shatters perceptions and expectations we and others may have had, but learning that our biological sex is the opposite from what we thought it was has an impact on our sexual orientation and relationships with others.

Furthermore, just because DSD male athletes have a natural sporting advantage, it doesn't mean that they haven't worked as hard as female athletes. Should these athletes, at the height of their career, be reduced from a national hero to some kind of a "cheat", and their DSD diagnosis broadcast to the world?

Campaigners for the inclusion of trans-identifying male athletes harnessed this ethically sensitive situation to influence discourse around sex-segregation.

If a man is sufficiently "feminine" - for example if he has breasts and long hair, wears makeup and skirts, takes female hormones or uses a female name and female pronouns - then it would be "cruel" to not let him compete in a female category. After all, what female athletes and both feminine and feminised male athletes have in common, is that they cannot outcompete elite males. Therefore, the only chance these males have to compete at an elite level is if they are allowed to compete in a female category.

Are 46 XY DSD athletes biologically female?

In humans, sex is determined by the presence or absence of the Y chromosome. This is because all humans have an X chromosome in their genetic make up, but only males have a Y.

Normally, males have 46 XY karyotype, a penis, testicles and produce sperm, while females have a 46 XX karyotype, a vagina, uterus, ovaries and produce eggs. However, because the Y chromosome contains genetic information necessary for the embryo to develop into a male, even individuals with atypical karyotypes such as 47 XXY, 47 XYY or 49 XXXXY will be male, while 47 XXX or 45 X0 individuals will be female.

There are many different genetic abnormalities that can give rise to Disorders of Sex Development (DSD). Sometimes, genes on the Y chromosome - such as the SRY gene which is involved in the development of testicles - can be deleted or even "jump" onto the X. Or genes on sex chromosomes or autosomes, which play a part in sex differentiation, can mutate. One of these genes is an androgen receptor gene which is found on the X chromosome and mutations can result in partial or complete androgen insensitivity (PAIS and CAIS). Very rarely, DSDs can also arise when two or more fertilised cells merge during very early development. As a result, the person has multiple karyotypes throughout their body, and this can mean a mixture of male and female cell lines (Dumic, et al., 2008).

As a consequence of these genetic abnormalities the developing embryo can receive erroneous signals, or fail to receive appropriate ones, and subsequently develop ambiguous genitalia, some opposite sex reproductive structures or absent or non-functional gonads, and in some cases, a male body could feminise while a female body could masculinise.

Traditionally, it was assumed that embryonic development is sex-neutral until gonads (ovaries or testes) start to develop and secrete sex hormones, which directs the body's development down the sex-appropriate pathway. However, if a male foetus is resistant to testosterone, or it fails to masculinise for some other reason (or if a female foetus inappropriately masculinises) the genetic sex of such an individual will be at odds with their appearance (phenotype).

Because our external appearance drives both self-perception and how others see us, 46 XY DSD males with a female phenotype typically have a female gender identity and are socially considered to be women, while 46 XX DSD females with a male phenotype typically have a male gender identity and are considered to be men.

This mismatch between genotype and phenotype, as well as other sex ambiguities, gave rise to the myth that people with DSDs are "intersex" (between male and female), that they are "hermaphrodites" (both male and female), or "pseudohermaphrodites" (an outdated medical term for a mismatch between external genitalia and gonads). It also led to claims such as "sex is a spectrum" and that a 46 XY person can be "female but maybe not 100%".

However, in recent years it has been shown that sex chromosomes start to drive sex differentiation soon after fertilisation -

way before gonads or sex hormones appear - and this affects all tissues in the body, including bones, muscles, blood, heart, lungs, liver, brain and so on (Deegan & Engel, 2019; Lowe, et al., 2015; Heydari, et al., 2022).

This means that male-female sex differences are more fundamental than just physical appearance, gonads and sex hormones. They exist on a genetic and molecular level, are driven by different sex chromosome complements - X and Y for male, only X for female - and they produce physiological differences that explain why 46 XY DSD athletes have a male sporting advantage, despite incomplete masculinisation.

The way forward

Male sporting advantage is so significant, that even the arguably greatest female athlete of all time, Serena Williams, could not beat male tennis player Karsten Braach, whose ATP ranking was World No. 203 at the time of the match. Serena didn't lose because she was a worse player. In fact she was much better, considering her outstanding successes in female competition. However, Braach was naturally stronger, faster and taller, which determined how hard he was able to hit the ball, reach far ends of the court and stretch to return. This natural physical advantage alone allowed him to beat the best female player at the height of her career.

Another example is the famous doubles match in the final of 1977 US Open, when Martina Navratilova and Betty Stöve played Ann Grub Stuart and Renee Richards. Richards is a biological male who underwent gender reassignment as an adult. The fact that Martina and her partner won is often used by transactivists to claim that the inclusion of normally sexed males won't necessarily come at the expense of fair play for women.

However, at the time of this match, Richards was 43 years old, which was 22 years older than Navratilova. Imagine if Richards entered women's tennis in their youth, and played against elite females of the same age. The female players would not stand a chance.

As we saw at the 2016 Rio Olympics, the inclusion of DSD males in female sport can have much the same effect. Even with testosterone suppression rules in place - because they neither apply to all events nor fully mitigate male sporting advantage - biologically male athletes are outperforming biological females in many events, and now the testosterone suppression requirement has been removed by the IOC altogether.

In my opinion, forcing DSD male athletes to undergo surgical procedures or take drugs they don't need, in order to be eligible to compete with females, is as antithetical to the ethics of sport as doping. Therefore I support the rejection of testosterone suppression rules. However, addressing the unfairness toward DSD males, without addressing the unfairness toward female athletes, is not going to work in the long term.

Furthermore, with transactivism conflating DSD and transgender in order to normalise the feminisation of males and masculinisation of females with hormones and surgery, it is only a matter of time before males who were gender-reassigned at the onset of puberty start entering female competitions. There hasn't been such a case yet, but to make an educated guess, their sporting advantage will at least be comparable to DSD males.

How will females who had undergone gender reassignment as minors and had their bodies masculinised compare to the feminised males? How will these females compare to normally sexed male athletes, considering that despite hormonal manipulation, their lack of a Y chromosome means that they can never attain the male sporting advantage?

Under femininity-based inclusion rules, it is likely that gender-reassigned females will be excluded on account of taking masculinising doses of testosterone, while feminised males will be permitted to compete in female sport. This might seem far-fetched now, but even if the practice of gender reassignment was to stop tomorrow, enough children have already been affected that we must anticipate this becoming an issue in the future.

The reality is that both trans-identifying and DSD males are currently competing in the wrong sex category. Acknowledging this needn't affect the social convention of referring to DSD males as "women". However, there are areas where biological sex is relevant - and sport is one of those.

Male advantage of course depends on the sport, but regardless of whether the advantage is 10% or 50% it is insurmountable between opposite sex athletes of the same age and fitness level. In elite sport, there are only so many places on the team and on the podium. While the predicament of males who, for one reason or another, cannot compete in elite male sport rightfully evokes compassion, I would like the world to show the same compassion for females too.

Female athletes have fought long and hard against prejudice and discrimination borne from their competitive disadvantage in relation to males. They have been ogled, infantilised, underfunded, sabotaged and sexually assaulted because of their female sex, by those of the male sex. Although these issues have, in some cases, affected biological males with a feminine appearance, I don't believe this is a sufficient reason to justify making female sport a mixed-sex category.

I would like to reiterate that DSD males and trans-identifying males are not the same. They are different biologically and they face very different challenges. However, for the purposes of inclusion in female sport, the two are related in practice, if not in spirit, and ultimately female athletes pay the price.

Women and girls are half the population and they deserve to compete fairly. We also have hopes and dreams of standing on the podium, proving our worth, getting sponsorships, or scholarships, prize money and a career in sport. Our self-esteem, sense of self and future prospects are all affected by the way current rules prioritise male inclusion over fair play for women and girls. I am here to ask that our human right of having access to single-sex spaces, which by definition includes female-only sport, is respected. Without exception.

Bibliography

Elsas, L.J. Ljungqvist, A. Ferguson-Smith, M.A. Simpson, J.L. Genel, M. Carlson, A.S. Ferris, E. de la Chapelle, A. Ehrhardt, A.A. (2000). Gender verification of female athletes. Genetics in Medicine. July-Aug Vol 2. No 4. https://www.nature.com/articles/gim2000258.pdf?origin=ppub

Marta, C.C. Marinho, D.A. Barbosa, T.M. Izquierdo, M. Marques, M.C. (2012). Physical fitness differences between prepubescent boys and girls. Journal of strength and conditioning research, 26(7), 1756–1766. https://doi.org/10.1519/JSC.0b013e31825bb4aa

Ferguson-Smith, M.A. Bavington, L.D. (2014). Natural Selection for Genetic Variants in Sport: The Role of Y Chromosome Genes in Elite Female Athletes with 46,XY DSD. Sports Med 44, 1629–1634 (2014). https://doi.org/10.1007/s40279-014-0249-8

International Olympic Committee. (2015). IOC consensus meeting on sex reassignment and hyperandrogenism. https://stillmed.olympic.org/Documents/Commissions_PDFfiles/Medical_commission/2015-11_ioc_consensus_meeting_on_sex_reassignment_and_hyperandrogenism-en.pdf

Mokgadi Caster Semenya v. International Association of Athletics Federation. (2018). Court of Arbitration for Sport. CAS 2018/O/5794 & 5798. https://www.tas-cas.org/fileadmin/user_upload/CAS_Award_-_redacted_-_Semenya_ASA_IAAF.pdf

Ingle, S. (2019). Caster Semenya accuses IAAF of using her as a 'guinea pig experiment'. https://www.theguardian.com/sport/2019/jun/18/caster-semenya-iaaf-athletics-guinea-pig

Dunbar, G. Imray, G. (2020). Semenya loses at Swiss supreme court over testosterone rules. https://apnews.com/article/switzerland-track-and-field-archive-courts-caster-semenya-bd69bc7ea983d9a1959813402d3d3472

Hilton, E.N. Lundberg, T.R. Transgender Women in The Female Category of Sport: Is the Male Performance Advantage Removed by Testosterone Suppression?. Preprints 2020, 2020050226 (doi: 10.20944/preprints202005.0226.v1). https://www.preprints.org/manuscript/202005.0226/v1

Ralph, J. (2017). Transgender footballer Hannah Mouncey waits on AFLW draft ruling. https://archive.md/olg1R

Presley, R. (2021). Transgender MMA Fighter Fallon Fox Breaks Opponent's Skull. https://www.attacktheback.com/transgender-mma-fighter-fallon-fox-breaks-opponents-skull/

World Rugby, (2021). Transgender Guidelines. https://www.world.rugby/the-game/player-welfare/guidelines/transgender

FPFW, (2021). Who should be competing for female medals at Tokyo 2020? Fair Play For Women. https://fairplayforwomen.com/laurel_hubbard/

Lohn, J. (2022). Lia Thomas Saga: With NCAA Championships Now Here, Betrayal of Female Athletes Continues. https://www.swimmingworldmagazine.com/news/as-ivy-league-champs-approach-conference-and-penn-have-betrayed-women-during-lia-thomas-controversy/

Lord, C. (2022). Indecent Exposure Laws Cited In Letter To U.S. Legal Authorities Highlights Litigation Threat To Sports & College Bosses Blind To Women's Rights In Transgender Debate. https://www.stateofswimming.com/indecent-exposure-laws-cited-in-letter-to-u-s-legal-authorities-highlights-litigation-threat-to-sports-college-bosses-blind-to-womens-rights-in-transgender-debate/

Rushing, E. (2022). 16 Penn swimmers send letter saying teammate Lia Thomas has an unfair advantage. The Philadelphia Enquirer. https://www.inquirer.com/college-sports/lia-thomas-penn-swimming-opposition-letter-20220204.html

International Olympic Committee. (2021). IOC framework on fairness, inclusion and non-discrimination on the basis of gender identity and sex variations. https://stillmed.olympics.com/media/Documents/News/2021/11/IOC-Framework-Fairness-Inclusion-Non-discrimination-2021.pdf?ga=2.195521836.1048075235.1637092563-834742310.1637092563

Dumic, M. Lin-Su, K. Leibel, N. I. Ciglar, S. Vinci, G. Lasan, R. Nimkarn, S. Wilson, J. D. McElreavey, K. & New, M. I. (2008). Report of fertility in a woman with a predominantly 46,XY karyotype in a family with multiple disorders of sexual development. The Journal of Clinical Endocrinology and Metabolism, 93(1), 182–189. https://doi.org/10.1210/jc.2007-2155

Deegan, D.F. Engel, N. (2019). Sexual Dimorphism in the Age of Genomics: How, When, Where. Front. Cell Dev. Biol., 06 September 2019. https://doi.org/10.3389/fcell.2019.00186

Lowe, R. Gemma, C. Rakyan, V. K. & Holland, M. L. (2015). Sexually dimorphic gene expression emerges with embryonic genome activation and is dynamic throughout development. BMC genomics, 16(1), 295. https://doi.org/10.1186/s12864-015-1506-4

Heydari, R. Jangravi, Z. Maleknia, S. Seresht-Ahmadi, M. Bahari, Z.

Salekdeh, G.H. Meyfour, A. (2022). Y chromosome is moving out of sex determination shadow. Cell Biosci. 2022 Jan 4;12(1):4. doi: 10.1186/s13578-021-00741-y. PMID: 34983649; PMCID: PMC8724748. https://cellandbioscience.biomedcentral.com/articles/10.1186/s13578-021-00741-y

Chapter 19

How Did Medical Institutions Get Captured by Gender Identity Ideology?

One of the transactivists' most persuasive arguments is that the entire medical profession agrees that sex is a spectrum, that our internal sense of "gender identity" - rather than our biological sex - determines whether we are male or female and that humans can change sex.

Although they cannot provide actual scientific evidence to support these claims, transactivists point to the practices of gender self-identification and the "affirmation approach" to treating gender dysphoria.

The supposed "sex change" involves anything from declaring the opposite sex gender identity, changing the name, pronouns, and dress style to that associated with the opposite sex, to medical and surgical body modification. This process is supported administratively by allowing individuals to change their sex markers on official documents and facilitating access to spaces reserved for the opposite sex, such as medical wards, toilets, prisons, and sports.

Wherever you turn, from the National Health Service

(NHS), General Medical Council (GMC), Royal Medical Colleges, Royal College of Nursing (RCN) and Nursing and Midwifery Council (NMC) to the British Psychological Society (BPS) and other allied fields, healthcare institutions have enthusiastically conflated sex and gender, implemented gender self-identification in their policies and all but stopped collecting accurate data on whether service users are male or female. This ideological and pseudoscientific shift has not only compromised patient care, it has come at the expense of women's sex-based rights as well as child safeguarding.

The problems these policies have created for healthcare practitioners, and their ability to carry out their duties ethically and professionally, have been meticulously analysed in a document entitled "Nurses request that health and nursing organisations withdraw from Stonewall's Diversity Championship Scheme" (Helyar, et al., 2021). In this document, the authors raised ethical and safety concerns regarding puberty blockers and cross-sex hormones for minors diagnosed with gender dysphoria. They also detailed the extent to which the NHS Trusts have chosen to defy the NHS Pledge, the CQC Guidance to Providers, and the single-sex exemptions under the Equality Act 2010 (all of which provide for single-sex accommodation and services in healthcare settings), in order to cater to the demands of gender self-identification lobbyists.

For example, in their 'Gender Reassignment Policy', NHS Greater Glasgow and Clyde present a hypothetical scenario where a female patient complains about the presence of a man who identifies as a woman, on what is supposed to be a women-only hospital ward. In such a case, the Trust instructs nurses to "re- iterate that the ward is indeed female-only and that there are no men present" (NHS Greater Glasgow and Clyde, 2018).

Some Trusts allow male sex offenders who identify as

women to be placed on women's wards (Nottinghamshire Healthcare NHS Foundation Trust, 2018; Oxford Health NHS Foundation Trust, 2019; Devon Partnership NHS Trust, 2018).

Nottinghamshire Trust even warns their staff that they should be "very careful if deciding to refuse...Just bear in mind you would be in more trouble for denying someone's rights!", while Devon Trust indicates that long-term segregation and seclusion might be appropriate for female patients who object to the Trust's gender self-identification policy.

Throughout the NHS, men who identify as women are accommodated on wards that correspond "to their gender presentation". In reality, only self-declaration is required, because trans-identifying people are accommodated according to their wishes, regardless of whether they have commenced "gender transition" at all.

Many Trusts that allow gender self-identification also redefine the protected characteristic of "sex" as either "gender" or "gender identity" (neither of which are protected characteristics or clearly defined in law), and they liken women's objection to the presence of male patients on women's wards to "racism" (Humber NHS Foundation Trust, 2018).

These policies appear to have been written around the same time, 2018-2019, and the same language and talking points can be seen throughout. Another thing they have in common is a lack of evidence that the impact of these policies on other protected characteristics - such as sex, age, disability, or religion - has ever been adequately assessed.

This echoes the circumstances surrounding the Annex B part of the NHS policy "Delivering same-sex accommodation for trans people and gender variant children" (NHS England and NHS Improvement, 2019).

As with other NHS policies that legitimise gender self-identification in healthcare settings, Annex B doesn't appear to have been subject to adequate consultation or impact assessment. Despite this, Annex B is being used to drive gender self-identification policies throughout the UK medical establishment.

It's worth noting that hospital accommodation policies are only one part of a much bigger problem. We have witnessed the rapid replacement of biological sex with self-identified gender on patient forms, which inform us that "female" now includes "women and trans women" - the latter being biological males - while "male" now includes "men and transmen" - the latter being biological females. This has effectively replaced single-sex data with mixed-sex data, and enabled widespread and unmonitored mis-sexing of patients in healthcare settings.

The new rules also allow both patients and doctors to self-identify as the opposite sex and to scrub their new records of any evidence of their actual sex.

More disturbing, perhaps, is the deliberate dissociation of female biology from words such as "female", "woman" and "mother", while the words "man" and "male" remain unaffected. Testicular cancer and prostate screening still affect "men", but to say that cervical cancer affects women is "exclusionary". Women have become "people with a cervix", "menstruators" and "vulva-owners". Maternity wards speak of "pregnant people" and even "birthing bodies" and the word "mother" is increasingly being portrayed as "trans-exclusionary" while the word "father" is, apparently, fine.

Concerned doctors, nurses, and patients have tried on many occasions to find out who decided, and on what basis, to replace biological sex with self-identified gender identity in healthcare settings. There is no other area where biological sex is more relevant to the needs and outcomes of service users, so the sudden realisation that our healthcare institutions have disregarded this basic fact was shocking. I think I can speak for many of us when I say that we assumed that alternative mechanisms were put in place to ensure that patients aren't mis-sexed and to safeguard female patients from indignities and assaults they are vulnerable to in mixed-sex healthcare settings. However, we were wrong, and when we raised the alarm, it fell on deaf ears.

We found that the GMC supports gender self-identification (GMC, no date), as does NHS England, which uses Annex B to justify similar policies.

The Royal Medical Colleges and companies that insure doctors, such as The Medical Protection Society (MPS) and the Medical Defense Union (MDU), point to the GMC guidance when they are now routinely advising concerned doctors to just go along with this.

It doesn't seem to matter how serious our concerns are; whether they are about child trafficking that could be facilitated by changing a child's sex marker and NHS number on request or the potential misuse of gender self-identification by male sex offenders. Disregarded, too, are the instances where male patients have already self-identified as women, gained access to women's wards and assaulted female patients.

The medico-legal advice seems to rely on the pointing circle between the NHS, GMC and the Royal Colleges, and the outcome is a slew of nearly-identical policies that have disregarded UK law, scientific facts and the safety of the vulnerable. This has been done in order to facilitate male access to female-only spaces. I specifically wish to highlight this consequence of gender self-identification, because although some females are accessing male-only facilities, as well, they make themselves vulnerable by doing so. This is obvious given that over 90% of sexual assaults are committed by men and the vast majority of victims are women. Authorities already know about the specific risks of male violence towards women and policies such as those regulating prison accommodation highlight this; women who self-identify as men are not being transferred to the male estate due to the high risk of violence toward them. However, men who self-identify as women are routinely transferred to the female estate, where some of them have raped and assaulted female inmates. Therefore, the encroachment on opposite sex spaces is mostly carried out by men and it is their access to female facilities that is the main focus of transactivist efforts, as well as the source of this movement's greatest controversy.

Two-pronged attack on the reality of biological sex

The replacement of sex with gender identity in healthcare policies is the end result of the medical experimentation on gender non-conforming people, as well as the outcome of a decades-long international campaign for "transgender rights". A thorough exploration of these topics is unfortunately beyond the scope of this book. So with that in mind, I would like to use a non-exhaustive list of examples to broadly illustrate how this radical and ill-advised change was achieved.

The practice of gender reassignment started with medical experiments at the turn of the 20th century. These experiments were initially designed to "cure" same-sex attraction and, failing that, to "convert" same-sex attracted people into heterosexual people of the opposite sex. Historically, a variety of methods were employed, depending on the sex of the patient. Men had ovaries and uteruses sown into their abdominal cavities in order to "turn them into women", they were castrated and had their penises removed and replaced with surgically constructed "artificial vaginas". Women had their breasts, ovaries and uteruses removed, and had artificial "phalluses" fashioned using skin and muscle from other parts of their bodies.

When these experiments first started, they were considered "ethical" due to the prominence of eugenics and homophobia at the time, which called for people who suffered from so-called "abnormal inversion of sexual attraction" to be sterilised. These experiments, as well as the forced sterilisations of gender non-conforming people, continued under the Nazi regime, and after the Second World War.

The practice of gender reassignment as we know it today, was developed in the 1960s by Alfred Kinsey, John Money and Harry Benjamin, who believed that "gender identity" - or our internal sense of being male or female - was socially constructed and therefore malleable. To this end, they used sex hormones, hormone blockers, cosmetic surgery and psychotherapy to change the appearance and "gender identity" of children with atypical genitalia, as well as adults who wanted to appear as the opposite sex.

The most famous centre that offered these procedures was Johns Hopkins Hospital, which ran the "sex change" programme between 1965 and 1979. When this was shut down, amid growing concerns that there was little evidence of long-term benefit and increasing evidence of harm, the Harry Benjamin International Gender Dysphoria Association was formed. This group of mostly therapists, psychologists and others who declared an interest in transgenderism, used Harry Benjamin's cases to devise Standards of Care for the treatment of gender dysphoria.

Meanwhile in the UK, patients had started campaigning for single-sex NHS wards, in order to reduce the risk of men sexually assaulting women in hospital, and to respect the privacy and dignity of patients of both sexes. These efforts were at odds with the ongoing push by transgender activists to be treated for all purposes as the members of the opposite sex.

One of the most notable lobbying and legal advice organisations for transgender people was Press for Change, who have worked with the UK government on many key pieces of legislation, including the Gender Recognition Act 2004 (GRA).

The GRA enshrined the legal fiction that humans can change sex into law. It did this by allowing transsexuals to change the sex markers on their birth certificates, which allowed transsexuals to marry their same-sex partners at a time when same-sex marriage was still illegal.

Women's groups were not consulted about the GRA, even though serious concerns about the impact of this law on women's sex-based rights were raised during Parliamentary debates (FPFW, 2018 (1); FPFW, 2018 (2); @HairyLeggdHarpy, 2018). Instead, it was argued that with only a few thousand individuals across the UK fulfilling the criteria for a Gender Recognition Certificate (such as having a medical diagnosis of Gender Identity Disorder and evidence of living in the "opposite sex role" for two years), the new legislation would not significantly impact women's sex-based rights.

Then, in 2006, a group of human rights lawyers put together a legally non-binding document entitled *The Yogyakarta Principles*, which outlined the application of international human rights law in relation to sexual orientation and gender identity. Although this document discussed many important issues affecting same-sex attracted and gender non-conforming people, it prioritised gender identity over sex, redefined same-sex attraction as "attraction to the same gender", and promoted the practice of gender self-identification (The Yogyakarta Principles, 2007; Harrison, 2018).

One of the co-authors and signatories to this document was a veteran transgender rights campaigner and a Professor of Equalities Law, Stephen Whittle.

Whittle came out as a "female to male" (FTM) transsexual in 1974, after returning from the Women's Liberation Conference in Edinburgh, which Whittle attended as a member of the Manchester Lesbian Collective. In 1975, Whittle started taking cross-sex hormones and soon after joined support groups for transsexuals, founding the FTM Network in 1989.

In 1992, Whittle co-founded Press for Change which led the campaign for full legal recognition for transgender people in the UK, which culminated in the passing of the Gender Recognition Act 2004.

Whittle underwent surgical gender reassignment between 2001 and 2003 and married their long-term female partner in 2005. The same year, Whittle was awarded an Officer of the Order of the British Empire (OBE) "for services to Gender Issues" (Wikipedia, no date (1)).

In 2007, the Harry Benjamin International Gender Dysphoria Association was renamed the World Professional Association for Transgender Health (WPATH), and Stephen Whittle became its President.

Another transactivist who, like Whittle, worked with both Press for Change and WPATH is Christine Burns, a trans-identifying male IT consultant and a Tory activist (LinkedIn, no date; LGBT History Month, 2005).

Burns joined Press for Change in 1993, came out as transgender in 1995, and acted as one of the principal negotiators between Press for Change and the UK government Ministers during the drafting and debating of the Gender Recognition Bill (McNab, 2000).

A particularly passionate advocate of the position that "trans women are women", Burns has criticised feminists who advocated for female-only rape crisis centres, going as far as to say, "In a bizarre way rapists have a better line in manners. At least they treat their victims, without prejudice, as women" (Burns, 1996).

Following the successful passing of the GRA2004, Burns was awarded a Member of the Most Excellent Order of the British Empire (MBE) "for services to Gender Issues" and moved into trans health advocacy.

After Press for Change successfully lobbied the Department of Health to rename the Sexual Orientation Advisory Group (SOAG) to the Sexual Orientation and Gender Identity Advisory Group (SOGIAG) in 2005, Burns became a chair of its transgender workstream. In this capacity, Burns commissioned various publications, including guidance for GPs. Burns also authored a resource for NHS managers and policymakers titled "Trans: A Practical Guide for the NHS" (Department of Health, 2008) and invited Charing Cross Gender Identity Clinic into discussions at the Parliamentary Forum on Transsexualism.

The following year, Burns was formally appointed to DoH LGBT Advisory Group' (Department of Health, 2009 (1)). Burns continued to be involved with the NHS through consulting on several NHS Northwest projects, becoming the programme manager for its Equality and Diversity Team in 2009 (Burns, 2010) and authoring a variety of LGBT resources, including a GP benchmarking tool titled 'Pride in Practice' (The Lesbian and Gay Foundation, 2011).

In 2010, Burns was appointed a co-chair of the LGBT Health Summit - a yearly event that brought together community organisers, healthcare, voluntary and statutory sector professionals and grassroots transactivists.

Subsequently, Burns was recognised by WPATH for "leadership and knowledge of trans people in healthcare" and invited to represent the UK on WPATH's international advisory panel

(WPATH, 2012). This panel influenced the *Standards of Care for the Health of Transsexual, Transgender, and Gender Nonconforming People Version 7* and made advisory input to the WPATH submission to the International Classification of Diseases revision process in the World Health Organisation (Wikipedia, no date (2)).

WPATH married the medical practice of gender reassignment with political activism for transgender rights, and has been instrumental in promoting gender self-identification and gender reassignment practices to medical institutions around the world. This has resulted in the medical implications of gender reassignment interventions, as well as gender self-identification, being filtered through the lens of transgender activism.

For example, long-term follow up studies have demonstrated that the majority of children who previously identified as the opposite sex would desist as long as they were left unmedicated. They often simply grew up to become well-adjusted same-sex attracted adults (Singh, et al., 2021; also see Detransition data in References section of essay number 10).

On the other hand, the studies on long-term outcomes following medical gender reassignment showed increased mortality, morbidity and suicide compared to non-reassigned cohorts (Dhejne, et al., 2011).

Despite this, WPATH decided to endorse poor quality studies that relied on a small number of patients, a lack of controls, a lack of long-term follow-up and a peer review process carried out by their own journal Transgender Health. They then used this "evidence" to convince medical institutions, as early as 2009, to adopt the experimental practice of validating opposite-sex identities in minors through the use of puberty blockers, cross-sex hormones and "gender affirming" surgeries (Hembree, et al., 2009). This "affirmative approach" to gender dysphoria has become a mandatory practice in many centres, despite the wider medical community never being consulted.

Around the same time in the UK - where it looked like the campaign for single-sex NHS wards would finally come to fruition - a letter titled "Eliminating Mixed Sex Accommodation" written by the Chief Nursing Officer and Director General NHS Finance, Performance and Operations, was circulated to the NHS Trusts. Although the letter claimed to "support the NHS commitment to providing every patient with same-sex accommodation, helping to safeguard their privacy and dignity when they are often at their most vulnerable", in the section titled "Annex E - Delivering same-sex accommodation for trans people and gender variant children" - it stated:

"Transsexual people, that is, individuals who have proposed, commenced or completed reassignment of gender, enjoy legal protection against discrimination. In addition, good practice requires that clinical responses be patient-centred, respectful and flexible towards all transgender people who do not meet these criteria but who live continuously or temporarily in the gender role that is opposite to their natal sex. General key points are that:

- Trans people should be accommodated according to their presentation: the way they dress, and the name and pronouns that they currently use.
- This may not always accord with the physical sex appearance of the chest or genitalia;
- It does not depend upon their having a gender recognition certificate (GRC) or legal name change;
- It applies to toilet and bathing facilities (except, for instance, that pre-operative trans people should not share open shower facilities);

- Views of family members may not accord with the trans person's wishes, in which case, the trans person's view takes priority.

Those who have undergone full-time transition should always be accommodated according to their gender presentation. Different genital or breast sex appearance is not a bar to this, since sufficient privacy can usually be ensured through the use of curtains or by accommodation in a single side room adjacent to a gender appropriate ward. This approach may only be varied under special circumstances where, for instance, the treatment is sex-specific and necessitates a trans person being placed in an otherwise opposite gender ward. Such departures should be proportionate to achieving a 'legitimate aim', for instance, a safe nursing environment" (Department of Health, 2009 (2)).

The language here, and especially the mention of a "legitimate aim", appears to address the wording in the Equality Act, which was passed by the UK Parliament the following year. This Act advises that transgender individuals may lawfully be *excluded* from opposite sex facilities despite their gender self-identification, if it is a "proportionate means to achieving a legitimate aim" such as would be the case in delivering same-sex healthcare facilities and services.

However, the GRA2004 never having emphasised the limitations of the legal fiction on which it relied, combined with the widespread belief in the NHS and the government that undergoing - or proposing to undergo - gender reassignment constituted "sex change" and legally entitled individuals to unrestricted access to opposite-sex spaces, meant that the single-sex exemptions as outlined in the EA2010 could not be enforced.

Consequently, when the UK government pledged to end

mixed-sex hospital accommodation in August 2010 (BBC, 2010), they did not remove Annex E from the NHS policy. This ensured that hospital accommodation remained mixed-sex due to the inclusion of individuals who self-identified as the opposite sex (Harper-Wright, 2018).

The next step toward gender self-identification was to "de-pathologise" the mental distress associated with the belief that one was "born in the wrong body".

To this end, the diagnosis of Gender Identity Disorder was replaced with Gender Dysphoria in 2013 and, seemingly overnight, it had become unacceptable to acknowledge any meaningful similarities between the transgender phenomenon and other related mental health conditions, such as Anorexia Nervosa, Body Integrity Identity Disorder and Body Dysmorphic Disorder. Instead, the focus was shifted to society's unwillingness to go along with one's self-perception.

In 2015, a veteran LGB charity which had close working relationships with all UK institutions, Stonewall UK, added the T (transgender) to their remit and started to campaign for gender self-identification. They additionally sought the review of the EA2010 "to include 'gender identity' rather than 'gender reassignment' as a protected characteristic and to remove exemptions, such as access to single-sex spaces" (Stonewall, 2015).

Soon afterwards, the LGBT Foundation successfully campaigned for the NHS HIV database to stop collecting information on patients' biological sex because it was "no longer best practice and probably illegal", and pushed instead for them to only collect data on self-identified gender (FPFW, 2021).

In 2017, ten more demands were added to *The Yogyakarta Principles*, the most relevant to sex-based rights and data collection being "Principle 31 - The Right to Legal Recognition", which states (emphasis mine):

"Everyone has the right to legal recognition without reference to, or requiring assignment or disclosure of, sex, gender, sexual orientation, gender identity, gender expression or sex characteristics. Everyone has the right to obtain identity documents, including birth certificates, regardless of sexual orientation, gender identity, gender expression or sex characteristics. *Everyone has the right to change gendered information in such documents while gendered information is included in them.*

STATES SHALL:

A. Ensure that official identity documents only include personal information that is relevant, reasonable and necessary as required by the law for a legitimate purpose, and thereby *end the registration of the sex and gender of the person in identity documents* such as birth certificates, identification cards, passports and driver licences, and as part of their legal personality;

B. Ensure access to a quick, transparent and accessible mechanism to change names, including to gender-neutral names, based on the self-determination of the person;

C. While sex or gender continues to be registered:

i. *Ensure a quick, transparent, and accessible mechanism that legally recognises and affirms each person's self-defined gender identity*;

ii. Make available a multiplicity of gender marker options;

iii. Ensure that no eligibility criteria, such as medical or psychological interventions, a psycho-medical diagnosis, minimum or maximum age, economic status, health, marital or parental status, or any other third party opinion, shall be a prerequisite to change one's name, legal sex or gender;

iv. *Ensure that a person's criminal record, immigration status or other status is not used to prevent a change of name, legal sex or gender.* (Yogyakarta Principles Plus 10, 2017).

Looking back on *The Yogyakarta Principles*, a signatory and

Professor of Human Rights Law, Robert Wintemute, said, "The issue of access to single-sex spaces largely affects women and not men. So it was easy for the men in the group to be swept along by a concern for LGBT rights and ignore this issue" (Bindel & Newman, 2021).

Be that as it may, the influence of this non-legally binding document on governments and medical establishments around the world has been profound. One after the other, the medical institutions, societies, and organisations brought their policies in line with its demands, and this was carried out behind the scenes and without widespread debates and consultations within the healthcare or legal professions.

Beliefs such as "born in the wrong body" were rewritten as fact, posited as true and authentic, and society's role in validating these beliefs was reformulated as therapeutic and a matter of basic human rights for trans-identifying people.

Debate about the ethics of such an approach was suppressed with the false suicide statistics associated with gender dysphoric young people (FPFW, 2018 (3)).

Anyone's unwillingness to use "preferred pronouns", any attempts to maintain single-sex spaces for women or, indeed, any societal resistance at all, was reframed by trans activists as "transphobia".

Eventually, one could no longer question the "affirmative approach" or any claims made by transactivists without being accused of "bigotry" and "wanting to harm trans people".

It is my sense that this two-pronged - medical and legal - approach was necessary because if someone objected to gender self-identification on legal grounds, they were told that the medical profession fully endorsed a "born in the wrong body" narrative as a factual, rather than metaphorical, phenomenon and that the "affirmative approach" orthodoxy was evidence of a biological basis for gender identity.

If the objections were based on scientific and medical grounds, such as the poor evidence-base for both gender identity and gender reassignment, or the reality that biological sex is binary and extremely important in the treatment of patients, they were told they were defying the law and denying transgender people's human rights.

Whichever way one turned, there were policies and pieces of legislation already in place that prevented institutions from critically examining the impact of gender self-identification on patients and society at large. That these policies and laws were brought in by stealth, and that they were demonstrably based on the erroneous basic premise - that humans can change sex and that gender identity overrides both sex and sexual orientation - did not seem to matter.

Luckily, since all these policies were "in advance of the law", following a titanic struggle by feminists, grassroots women's organisations, parents and conscientious professionals, the UK government eventually rejected proposals for gender self-identification.

Other countries were not so lucky.

In 2016, the outgoing US President Barack Obama redefined Title IX to prohibit discrimination on the basis of "gender identity", instead of its original intention to protect against discrimination based on sex. As a result, gender reassignment clinics have proliferated throughout the United States, and in 2021, the newly elected Biden administration passed an executive order prohibiting "discrimination on the basis of gender identity" which effectively replaced biological sex with self-identified gender in US law (Shaw, 2021).

Similar changes can be seen in Canada, Australia, New

Zealand, Ireland, India, and many other parts of the world. If gender self-identification isn't legal already, then transactivists are lobbying governments to make it so, while those who resist are censored, deplatformed, and maligned as "'TERFs", "transphobes," and "bigots".

The chilling effect of the emotional blackmail with false suicide statistics, as well as institutional capture by gender identity ideology, has resulted in an inability of the establishment to intervene in this evolving medical and social scandal.

The pushback

Radical feminists, such as Sheila Jeffreys, Germaine Greer and Dr Julia Long, have long recognised the negative impact men identifying as women have on women's rights, as well as lesbian and gay rights.

Women-only spaces became incredibly important during the second wave of feminist activism in the 1970s and it was the exclusion of males that enabled women to safely share their experiences of male violence with one another and gave them room to organise to counteract the effects of patriarchal oppression. Women fundraised and built safe spaces such as women-only restrooms, clubs and rape and domestic violence shelters. The forced inclusion of men in these safe spaces, which is the consequence of transgender activism, compromises the fragile protections women carved out for themselves in an otherwise male-dominated society.

The harms associated with gender reassignment experiments - especially those carried out on children with Disorders of Sex Development (DSDs) - were also substantially exposed in the late 1990s when one of the victims of these procedures, David Reimer, publicly recounted his ordeal. David, who was "reassigned to a girl" in infancy by John Money, and the team at Johns Hopkins Hospital, spoke of being abused and manipulated by John Money, alongside his twin brother Brian, and how "gender reassignment" interventions left him traumatised and struggling with mental health issues.

Having supported the unethical experiments with "sex reassignment" based on John Money's claims that the Reimer experiment had been a complete success, the medical establishment finally seemed to listen to patients who had been trying to raise awareness of the harms of these procedures.

Unfortunately, not long after the invasive procedures on DSD children fell out of favour, the practice was resurrected with a new cohort in mind - children who were diagnosed with gender dysphoria.

In the first decade of the 21st century, the media started embracing the narrative of "brave" parents allowing their children to cross-dress and to change their names and pronouns to the opposite sex. This was initially described as "gender-neutral parenting", a concept most liberal people could get behind. However, medical gender reassignment services soon started to experience a surge in referrals.

In 2009/2010, 32 girls and 40 boys were referred to the Tavistock Gender Identity Development Service (GIDS). In 2011/2012 the sex ratio flipped in favour of girls, and the number of referrals increased to 136. The referrals continued to rise and the sex ratio continued to widen year on year, until in 2016/2017, the total number of referrals reached 1981 children, with around 70% being adolescent girls (GIDS, 2021; Turner, 2022; Transgender Trend, 2019).

"Watchful waiting" once used to be the main approach to gender confused minors and resulted, overwhelmingly, in desistance. Now, though, children were being routinely puberty blocked, their bodies flooded with opposite-sex hormones and their healthy breasts and genitals surgically altered or removed. This was an approach that appeared to solidify opposite sex identification in the vast majority of children, cause iatrogenic harm and create life-long medical patients.

No explanation for this was forthcoming from the medical establishment, beyond vague claims that "better understanding of gender dysphoria" was driving both the surge in referrals and "affirmation" interventions. However, many in the medical and psychological community remained sceptical.

Why, in the age of the internet, the mainstreaming of pornography, and the surging sexual abuse in schools (Department of Education, 2021; Ferguson, 2021), might adolescent girls suddenly want to dis-identify with being female and wish to "become" male?

Troubled by these developments, an accomplished sculptor and communications expert Stephanie Davis Arai published the article "Is my child transgender?" on her parenting website in March 2015. In it, she critiqued the emerging practice of diagnosing children as "trans". In October 2015, her article "The Transgender Experiment on Kids" was published in The Wales Arts Review, and in November of the same year, her website Transgender Trend went live (Maynard, 2021).

In 2016, Dr Julia Long organised the "Thinking Differently - feminists questioning gender politics" conference in London, which aimed to "present a feminist critique of the politics and consequences of transgenderism and gender identity". Stephanie Davis Arai was invited to speak, alongside Sheila Jeffreys, Julie Bindel, Lierre Keith, Julia Long, Jackie Mearns, Mary Lou Singleton and Magdalen Berns.

In May 2017, Transgender Trend published *Is It Surprising That Referrals Of Children To The Tavistock Clinic Continue To*

Soar? Media Report 2016 – 17 (Transgender Trend, 2017), which was followed in early 2018 by *Transgender Trend - Resource Pack for Schools* (Transgender Trend, 2018).

On the other side of the Atlantic, in October 2017, Jungian analyst Lisa Marchiano published an article "Outbreak: On Transgender Teens and Psychic Epidemics" raising the possibility of social contagion driving the increase in trans-identification in children and young people (Marchiano, 2017).

Her concerns were echoed by Dr Lisa Littman in her seminal paper "Parent reports of adolescents and young adults perceived to show signs of a rapid onset of gender dysphoria" (Littman, 2018).

By 2017, there was already disquiet among therapists working for the Tavistock GIDS, many of whom voiced concerns about the lack of evidence-base, inadequate assessments, safeguarding failures and how transgender activists were driving the "affirmation approach".

In 2018, Tavistock governor and consultant psychiatrist Dr David Bell sent an internal report to service leaders at Tavistock, urging them to suspend all experimental hormone treatments for gender dysphoric children until there was better evidence of the outcomes (Bannerman, 2020).

In 2019, Dr Michael Biggs, an Associate Professor of Sociology at the University of Oxford, published a paper entitled "The Tavistock's Experiment with Puberty Blockers" (Biggs, 2019), where he analysed preliminary results of Tavistock's unpublished study and criticised the WPATH guidelines and medicalisation of gender-confused children.

That same year, tax expert and researcher on sustainable business and international development, Maya Forstater, lost an Employment Tribunal case against the Center for Global Development (CGD). She had commented on the impact gender identity ideology and gender self-identification are having on women's sex-based rights and as a consequence her contract with CGD was not renewed. She asserted that her belief that "sex is biological, binary, immutable and important" was covered by the protected characteristic "religion and belief" under section 10 of the Equality Act, and said that she "respected people's pronouns and rights to freedom of expression", but "enforcing the dogma that transwomen are women is totalitarian".

The Tribunal judge ruled that her beliefs were "incompatible with human dignity and fundamental rights of others" and were therefore not afforded protection under the Equality Act. He also claimed that her beliefs were "not worthy of respect in a democratic society", a characterisation typically applied to Holocaust denial and similarly dangerous beliefs (Maya Forstater vs CGD and others, 2019).

This decision caused outrage, prompting famous author JK Rowling to speak out on Maya's behalf. She tweeted: "Dress however you please. Call yourself whatever you like. Sleep with any consenting adult who'll have you. Live your best life in peace and security. But force women out of their jobs for stating that sex is real? #IStandWithMaya #ThisIsNotADrill" (JK Rowling, 2019).

Soon after, Maya Forstater announced that she would appeal the Tribunal judgement.

Despite the draconian policies that deemed any challenge to the affirmation-only approach an act of "transphobia", which was likely to instigate immediate disciplinary proceedings against the alleged offender, more and more clinicians spoke up. They wrote papers, open letters and rapid responses to articles promoting puberty blockers and cross-sex hormones for children, drawing attention to the poor evidence-base and potential harms.

In 2020, the Society for Evidence-Based Gender Medicine

(SEGM) was formed with an aim to provide summaries of evidence in this area, and to promote research and supportive psychosocial approaches for the care of young people with gender dysphoria.

Later that year, brave detransitioner Keira Bell, along with the mother of an autistic teen Mrs A, initiated a Judicial Review against Tavistock GIDS at the UK High Court. As a result of this review, which ruled in favour of Keira Bell and Mrs A (Quincy Bell and Mrs A vs The Tavistock and Portman NHS Foundation Trust, 2020), the prescription of puberty blockers for gender dysphoric children was halted. This was done amid concerns that the evidence-base for these treatments is lacking and that children cannot meaningfully consent to potentially serious and irreversible long-term side effects, such as sterility.

The concerns of the UK High Court were echoed in the systematic reviews of puberty blocker and cross-sex hormone treatments for children with gender dysphoria, which also urged caution due to the poor evidence-base (NICE, 2020 (1); NICE, 2020 (2)).

Tavistock GIDS appealed the High Court decision, and succeeded in overturning it on Appeal in 2021 (Bell and another vs The Tavistock and Portman NHS Foundation Trust and others, 2021). However, this judgement did not negate the findings of the original review regarding the appropriateness of these treatments.

Due to ongoing concerns in the medical profession, as well as the mainstream of society, the NHS commissioned an independent review into gender identity services for children and young people which was spearheaded by Dr Hilary Cass OBE. Dr Cass is a former President of the Royal College of Paediatrics and Child Health (NHSE, 2020).

Soon after, the Care and Quality Commission (CQC)

carried out an inspection at the Tavistock GIDS, where they identified significant concerns in areas of person-centred care, capacity and consent, safe care and treatment, governance as well as waiting times (CQC, 2021).

Internationally, Finland revised its guidelines to prioritise psychological support over medical interventions in June 2020, while in April 2021 the Karolinska Hospital, in Sweden, stopped prescribing puberty blockers and cross-sex hormones to gender dysphoric minors except in the context of clinical trials (SEGM, 2021).

In June 2021, the Maya Forstater judgement was overturned on appeal. The tribunal concluded that believing "biological sex is real, important and immutable" - which has since come to be known as "gender critical beliefs" - met the legal test of a "genuine and important philosophical position", and "could not be shown to be a direct attempt to harm others." Therefore, these beliefs were protected under the Equality Act 2010 and they "must be tolerated in a pluralist society" (Maya Forstater vs CGD and others, 2021).

The full merits hearing of Maya Forstater's Employment Tribunal case was held in March the following year where it was ruled that she was subjected to direct discrimination and victimisation because of her gender-critical beliefs (Maya Forstater vs CGD and others, 2022).

In late 2021 Sonia Appleby, a safeguarding lead at Tavistock and Portman NHS Trust, won an Employment Tribunal case against Tavistock GIDS. She showed that Tavistock had prevented her from carrying out her duties as a safeguarding lead, and subjected her to unfair disciplinary procedures after she brought forward the concerns of GIDS clinicians (BBC, 2021).

In February 2022, the Cass Review published an interim

report which echoed the concerns of dissenting clinicians and the wider public. The review also found that the evidence-base for the "affirmative approach" was lacking, that a more holistic and localised approach to the care of gender-questioning children is required and that gender identity services for children and young people needed to move from a single national provider to a regional model (The Cass Review, 2022; Cass, 2022).

In July 2022, NHS England announced that Tavistock GIDS would close by Spring 2023 (Hayward, 2022).

At the time of writing this essay there are ongoing attempts in many countries, including the US, New Zealand and Australia, to put the brakes on paediatric gender reassignment experiments. In my opinion, it is only a matter of time before gender self-identification and affirmation-only approach to gender dysphoria are exposed as the biggest medical and social scandals of our time.

Medical autonomy

Healthcare practitioners are ethically obliged to deliver safe and effective medical care. However, they are under enormous pressure from transactivists who demand that medical decisions are brought in line with gender identity ideology.

The medico-legal advice in this area is presented as "guidance" but uses prescriptive language. When this is combined with a culture of throwing false accusations of "transphobia" at anyone who raises objections to gender self-identification and affirmation-only practices, a busy practitioner might be tempted to go along with the demands of patients and transactivists, even when doing so conflicts with their clinical judgement.

One needs to only look at past medical scandals - from

Thalidomide and lobotomies, to symphysiotomies and forced sterilisations - to realise that harmful practices periodically come to thrive in the medical profession. It is important to remember, however, that medical ethics compels us to speak out against harmful treatments, regardless of how well embraced they might be by society and the medical establishment.

The GMC's "Good practice in prescribing and managing medicines and devices" states, "You are responsible for the prescriptions that you sign. You must only prescribe drugs when you have adequate knowledge of your patient's health. And you must be satisfied that the drugs serve your patient's need" (GMC, 2021).

Therefore, institutions can set guidelines, but doctors are, ultimately, responsible for their own prescribing and conduct. This is why the guidance regarding the prescribing of puberty blockers and cross-sex hormones is carefully couched in terms of recommendation and not instruction.

It is harder for doctors alone to resist policies that allow gender self-identification and the change of sex markers on personal documents, even though these policies negatively impact patient care due to the removal of single-sex accommodation and services in healthcare settings. In order to reverse these policies, institutions must painstakingly resolve their confusion about sex, gender, and the impact of gender self-identification on sex-based rights.

In any case, a doctor's primary obligation is to "First, do no harm". The benefits of proposed treatments have to outweigh the risks and they need to be backed by solid scientific rationale and good evidence. Patients need to be fully informed and competent to consent to all the possible outcomes, including complications and side effects. As long as these basic rules are respected, doctors have autonomy over their medical practice, including choosing not to facilitate treatments they believe to be harmful.

To give an example, some doctors are religious and morally against abortions. They believe that abortion amounts to the murder of a child and, in their worldview, the bodily autonomy of a mother does not trump the foetus' right to life. Ethically, denying a mother the right to bodily autonomy is not acceptable, so how can this be reconciled in clinical practice? Shaming and criticising the patient and deliberately impeding her access to abortion would breach medical ethics. Likewise, because doctors have autonomy too, the law can only ever grant patients the right to access abortion services; it cannot compel individual clinicians to provide these services. Therefore, the appropriate course of action would be for such a doctor to refer the patient seeking an abortion to a colleague willing to provide abortion care and counselling.

There's good evidence that abortions produce the desired results (termination of unwanted pregnancy) while having a low complication rate. Women require access to this treatment because the lack of access to abortion has caused much harm in the past.

Conversely, doctors who are refusing to participate in medical gender reassignment, by and large, are doing so not based on personal beliefs and morals but due to the lack of evidence of benefit and the mounting evidence of harm.

Medical gender reassignment has significant long-term side effects such as sterility, impairment of sexual and cognitive functions, bone mineralisation issues, and an increased cardiovascular risk in physically healthy yet psychologically distressed patients. Studies also show that, in the long-term, these treatments don't improve psychiatric outcomes (Hisle-Gorman, et al.,

2021; Van Mol et al, 2020; Alzahrani et al, 2019; Nota et al, 2019).

There is also a lack of randomised control trials and long-term follow-up in this area of medicine, and the loss to follow-up is unacceptably large.

In fact, The Royal College of General Practitioners (RCGP) has already criticised the "affirmation only" approach to treating gender dysphoria, and emphasised the importance of medical autonomy.

In their 2019 position statement, they reflected on the lack of robust and comprehensive evidence around the outcomes, side effects, and unintended consequences of medical gender reassignment, especially for children and young people, and pointed out that this prevents GPs from helping patients and their families to make informed decisions.

They also raised the issue of the impact of gender self-identification on patient care, particularly concerning sex-appropriate screening programmes, and highlighted conflicting advice the GMC gave regarding "bridging prescriptions" for patients who procured puberty blockers and cross-sex hormones on the internet.

On the one hand, the GMC advises GPs to undertake a harm-reduction strategy of prescribing bridging endocrine treatments to patients who are self-medicating with medicines bought on the internet or the black market. In this scenario, the GPs should seek advice from an experienced gender specialist and only prescribe these medicines if judged to benefit the patient overall.

On the other hand, the GMC "Good Medical Practice" ethical guidance states that GPs "must recognise and work within the limits of their competence".

Therefore, GPs are facing conflicting messages from their

regulator about how to approach and treat these patients. This poses significant medico-legal risks to GPs and compromises patient safety.

The RCGP concludes that "GPs are ultimately responsible for their prescribing and should not be pressured into prescribing where they feel it is unsafe or involves unacceptable risks. The GMC advice needs review and clarification." (RCGP, 2019)

As doctors, we are responsible for safeguarding our patients from malign political, ideological, and financial influences that might impact their medical treatment. Whenever the elite medical leadership abandons these principles, living up to this standard is more difficult for the individual clinician. However, this doesn't change medical ethics or our obligations.

It took minutes for anonymous bureaucrats to write gender identity ideology into medical policies and thousands of human hours to undo the damage. We are succeeding, but it is not over yet. The transgender lobby keeps coming up with new ways to coerce the medical profession to fulfil their demands, the latest being their cynical reframing of "watchful waiting" and talking therapies as "trans conversion therapy".

The Association of LGBTQ+ Doctors and Dentists (GLADD), for example, has recently published a "UK Medical Schools Charter on So-Called LGBTQ+' Conversion Therapy'", in which they ask medical schools to commit to "affirming LGBTQ+ people's gender and/or sexual identity". Most UK medical schools have signed it, and preferred pronouns appear alongside several signatures (@Rebecca35935662, 2022).

This is also being pushed through with the Conversion Therapy Ban Bill (UK Parliament, 2022). By including gender identity alongside sexual orientation, the Bill, which seeks to outlaw gay conversion therapy, may be used to mandate conversion therapy for another group - physically healthy gender dysphoric minors. Many of whom, as we already know, would most likely desist from opposite-sex identification and grow into healthy, often same-sex attracted, adults.

The transgender lobby seems to think they can use a combined medical and legal approach yet again to coerce clinicians to participate in medical gender reassignment, even though the harms of the "affirmation model" have become known in the mainstream, and patients are starting to sue their practitioners.

However, the unforeseen consequence, should the Conversion Therapy Ban Bill be made into law, could be that clinicians would consider it too medico-legally risky to accept gender dysphoric patients into their care.

So it seems that as a profession, we are at a crossroads.

I would like to conclude this essay with quotes from a paper entitled "When Psychiatry Battled the Devil", which analysed the Satanic ritual abuse scandal in the psychiatric profession.

"Some mass cultural phenomena are so emotionally charged, so febrile, and in retrospect so causally incomprehensible, that we feel compelled to move on silently and feign forgetfulness."

"Cautionary tales may prevent the recurrence of pyrogenic cultural fantasies and the devastating clinical mistakes they inspire."

"But who should tell this tale? To those of us who are old enough to have been there, that era already seems like a curious relic of the past, bracketed in our memory palaces behind a door we are loathe to open again." (Noll, 2013)

As clinicians, we need to openly and honestly examine the systemic failings which have caused us to stray away from the first principles of science and medicine and do our utmost to rectify them. If we don't, we risk repeating the same mistakes.

Bibliography

Helyar, S. Hill, A. Griffin, L. (2021). Nurses request that health and nursing organisations withdraw from Stonewall's Diversity Championship Scheme. https://lascapigliata.com/institutional-capture/nurses-request-that-health-and-nursing-organisations-withdraw-from-stonewalls-diversity-championship-scheme/

NHS Greater Glasgow and Clyde. (2018). Gender Reassignment Policy. https://drive.google.com/file/d/1wpSW6wpa-ka24dh9LqaqUM8qqAw96B8P/view

Nottinghamshire Healthcare NHS Foundation Trust. (2018). Trans Patients Policy and Procedure. https://drive.google.com/file/d/1rOxj6awoxvY9c_DIZb6lgDbyjYnYrXj6/view

Oxford Health NHS Foundation Trust. (2019). Supporting Transitioning Service Users Procedural Guidance. https://drive.google.com/file/d/1rxQSDjDH2q4QjAOUa6WpFi1kEpvEJ3ZA/view

Devon Partnership NHS Trust. (2018). Supporting Transgender, Non-Binary and Intersex Patients. https://drive.google.com/file/d/1RgVwdNTrd2TXaagibiCkkPNBujUN09_a/view

Humber NHS Foundation Trust. (2018). Policy for Supporting Transgender Patients N-060. https://drive.google.com/file/d/1T4tI0JdPsj1OuWPmhAVB5jrKnvCejRjU/view

NHS England and NHS Improvement. (2019). Delivering same-sex accommodation for trans people and gender variant children - Annex B. pp 12-14. https://www.england.nhs.uk/statistics/wp-content/uploads/sites/2/2021/05/NEW-Delivering_same_sex_accommodation_sep2019.pdf

GMC. (no date). Trans healthcare. https://www.gmc-uk.org/ethical-guidance/ethical-hub/trans-healthcare#Confidentiality%20and%20equality

FPFW. (2018 (1)). Transgender rights: How did we get here? Part 2: Changing legal sex status. Fair Play For Women. https://fairplayforwomen.com/transgender-rights-get-part-2-changing-legal-sex-status/

FPFW. (2018 (2)). Transgender rights: How did we get here? Part 1 Equality Law. Fair Play For Women. https://fairplayforwomen.com/transgender-rights-get-part-1-equality-law/

@HairyLeggdHarpy. (2018). Tweets from 2003: The Gender Recognition

Bill. https://web.archive.org/web/20191223045254/https:/twitter.com/HairyLeggdHarpy/status/1049289194370002945

The Yogyakarta Principles. (2007). https://www.oursplatform.org/wp-content/uploads/Yogyakarta-Principles-on-the-application-of-IHRL-to-SOGI.pdf

Harrison, H. (2018). Yogyakarta Principles: International Threat to Women's Rights. ObjectNow.org. https://objectnow.org/2018-7-27-yogyakarta-principles-international-threat-to-womens-rights/

Wikipedia. (no date (1)). Stephen Whittle. https://en.wikipedia.org/wiki/Stephen_Whittle

LinkedIn. (no date). Christine Burns. https://www.linkedin.com/in/christineburns

LGBT History Month. (2005). Christine Burns. https://web.archive.org/web/20160107162242/http://www.lgbthistorymonth.org.uk/documents/CBurnsOct2005.pdf

McNab, C. (2000). Government starts talking - Trans people meet the working group. https://www.webarchive.org.uk/wayback/archive/20060124120000/http://www.pfc.org.uk/news/2000/govtalk.htm

Burns, C. (1996). Safe for Some. https://web.archive.org/web/19991114012622/http://www.pfc.org.uk/gendrpol/safesome.htm

Department of Health. (2008). Trans: a practical guide for the NHS. https://webarchive.nationalarchives.gov.uk/ukgwa/20130123195237/http://www.dh.gov.uk/en/Publicationsandstatistics/Publications/PublicationsPolicyAndGuidance/DH_089941

Department of Health. (2009 (1)). Lesbian, Gay, Bisexual and Transgender Advisory Group. https://webarchive.nationalarchives.gov.uk/ukgwa/20100407212457/www.dh.gov.uk/en/Managingyourorganisation/Equalityandhumanrights/Sexualorientation/DH_4136008

Burns, C. (2010). The continued importance of Equality Impact Assessments. https://web.archive.org/web/20101122073058/http://help.northwest.nhs.uk/blog/2010/10/11/the-continued-importance-of-equality-impact-assessments/

The Lesbian and Gay Foundation. (2011). Pride in Practice. https://web.archive.org/web/20120210061051/http://www.lgf.org.uk/Our-services/pride-in-practice/7 (deleted page)

WPATH. (2012). International Advisory Group. https://web.archive.org/web/20121102053615/http://wpath.org/committees_international.cfm

Wikipedia. (no date (2)). Christine Burns. https://en.wikipedia.org/wiki/Christine_Burns

Singh, D. Bradley, S. Zucker, K. (2021). A Follow-Up Study of Boys With Gender Identity Disorder. frontiersin.org. https://www.frontiersin.org/articles/10.3389/fpsyt.2021.632784/full

Dhejne, C. Lichtenstein, P. Boman, M. Johansson, A.L.V. Långström, N. et al. (2011). Long-Term Follow-Up of Transsexual Persons Undergoing Sex Reassignment Surgery: Cohort Study in Sweden. PLOS ONE 6(2): e16885. https://doi.org/10.1371/journal.pone.0016885

Hembree, W. C. Cohen-Kettenis, P. Delemarre-van de Waal, H. A. Gooren, L. J. Meyer III, W. J. Spack, N. P. Tangpricha, V. Montori, V. M. (2009). Endocrine Treatment of Transsexual Persons: An Endocrine Society Clinical Practice Guideline. The Journal of Clinical Endocrinology & Metabolism, Volume 94, Issue 9, Pages 3132–3154. https://doi.org/10.1210/jc.2009-0345

Department of Health. (2009 (2)). Eliminating Mixed Sex Accommodation. https://assets.publishing.service.gov.uk/government/uploads/system/uploads/attachment_data/file/200215/CNO_note_dh_098893.pdf

BBC. (2010). Pledge to end mixed sex hospital accommodation. https://www.bbc.co.uk/news/health-10982566

Harper-Wright, A. (2018). Sex, Gender & the NHS Part 1: The "Single-Sex Hospital Wards" that have always been a lie. Medium. https://medium.com/@anneharperwright/sex-gender-the-nhs-1e8f4e6363a6

Stonewall. (2015). Women and Equalities Select Committee Inquiry on Transgender Equality. https://www.stonewall.org.uk/women-and-equalities-select-committee-inquiry-transgender-equality

FPFW. (2021). Why isn't the NHS collecting data on biological sex? https://fairplayforwomen.com/why-isnt-the-nhs-collecting-data-on-biological-sex/

The Yogyakarta Principles. (2017). The Yogyakarta Principles Plus 10. https://www.oursplatform.org/wp-content/uploads/YP-plus-10_Yogyakarta-Principles-Additional_2017.pdf

Bindel, J. Newman, M. (2021). The trans rights that trump all - Women's rights were not considered in legislation that allows trans people to effectively decide their own gender. https://thecritic.co.uk/issues/april-2021/the-trans-rights-that-trump-all/

FPFW. (2018 (3)) Trans suicide facts and myths. https://fairplayforwomen.com/suicide/

Shaw, D. (2021). Biden Administration Guts Female Rights Two Weeks After Dept of Ed Says Title IX Applies Only to Bio Sex. Women Are Human. https://www.womenarehuman.com/biden-administration-guts-female-rights-two-weeks-after-dept-of-ed-says-title-ix-applies-only-to-bio-sex/

GIDS. (2021). Referrals to GIDS, financial years 2010-11 to 2020-21. https://gids.nhs.uk/number-referrals

Turner, J. (2022). What Went Wrong at the Tavistock Clinic for Trans Teenagers? The Times. https://segm.org/GIDS-puberty-blockers-minors-the-times-special-report

Transgender Trend. (2019). The Surge in Referral Rates of Girls to the Tavistock Continues to Rise. https://www.transgendertrend.com/surge-referral-rates-girls-tavistock-continues-rise/

Department of Education. (2021). Sexual violence and sexual harassment between children in schools and colleges. https://assets.publishing.service.gov.uk/government/uploads/system/uploads/attachment_data/file/1014224/Sexual_violence_and_sexual_harassment_between_children_in_schools_and_colleges.pdf

Ferguson, D. (2021). Sexual abuse rife in UK's state and private schools, say police. The Guardian. https://www.theguardian.com/society/2021/mar/27/sexual-abuse-rife-in-state-schools-say-police

Maynard, L. (2021). Stephanie Davies-Arai & the story of Transgender Trend. https://lilymaynard.com/stephanie-davies-arai-transgender-trend/

Transgender Trend. (2017). Is It Surprising That Referrals Of Children To The Tavistock Clinic Continue To Soar? Media Report 2016 – 17. https://www.transgendertrend.com/surprising-referrals-children-tavistock-clinic-continue-soar/

Transgender Trend. (2018). Schools Resource Pack. https://www.transgendertrend.com/transgender-schools-guidance/

Marchiano, L. (2017) Outbreak: On Transgender Teens and Psychic Epidemics, Psychological Perspectives, 60:3, 345-366, https://doi.org/10.1080/00332925.2017.1350804

Littman L (2018) Parent reports of adolescents and young adults perceived to show signs of a rapid onset of gender dysphoria. PLoS ONE 13(8): e0202330. https://doi.org/10.1371/journal.pone.0202330

Bannerman, L. (2020). David Bell: Tavistock gender clinic whistleblower faces the sack. The Times. https://www.thetimes.co.uk/article/david-bell-tavistock-gender-clinic-whistleblower-faces-the-sack-rtkl09907

Biggs, M. (2019). The Tavistock's Experiment with Puberty Blockers. https://users.ox.ac.uk/~sfos0060/Biggs_ExperimentPubertyBlockers.pdf

Maya Forstater vs CGD and others (2019). The Employment Tribunal.

Case Number: 2200909/2019. 2019. https://assets.publishing.service.gov.uk/media/5e15e7f8e5274a06b555b8b0/Maya_Forstater__vs_CGD_Europe__Centre_for_Global_Development_and_Masood_Ahmed_-_Judgment.pdf

JK Rowling. (2019). Dress however you please. Call yourself whatever you like. Sleep with any consenting adult who'll have you. Live your best life in peace and security. But force women out of their jobs for stating that sex is real? #IStandWithMaya #ThisIsNotADrill Twitter. Dec 19, 2019. https://twitter.com/jk_rowling/status/1207646162813100033?lang=en

Quincy Bell and Mrs A vs The Tavistock and Portman NHS Foundation Trust. (2020). EWHC 3274 (Admin). Case No: CO/60/2020 https://www.judiciary.uk/wp-content/uploads/2020/12/Bell-v-Tavistock-Judgment.pdf

NICE. (2020 (1)). Evidence review: Gonadotrophin releasing hormone analogues for children and adolescents with gender dysphoria. https://drive.google.com/file/d/1jZ68aVpVkIlypnxIow36QYCNJtvT7tgp/

NICE. (2020 (2)). Evidence review: Gender-affirming hormones for children and adolescents with gender dysphoria. https://drive.google.com/file/d/1dp-H1A_eBwcGY9yuHdfPi77Wr5XlDNg1/

Bell and another vs The Tavistock and Portman NHS Foundation Trust and others. (2021). EWCA Civ 1363. Appeal No. C1/2020/2142 Case No: CO/60/2020. https://www.judiciary.uk/judgments/bell-and-another-v-the-tavistock-and-portman-nhs-foundation-trust-and-others/

NHSE. (2020). NHS announces independent review into gender identity services for children and young people. NHS England. https://www.england.nhs.uk/2020/09/nhs-announces-independent-review-into-gender-identity-services-for-children-and-young-people/

CQC. (2021). Care Quality Commission demands improved waiting times at Tavistock and Portman NHS Foundation Trust. Care Quality Commission. https://www.cqc.org.uk/news/releases/care-quality-commission-demands-improved-waiting-times-tavistock-portman-nhs

SEGM (2021.) Sweden's Karolinska Ends All Use of Puberty Blockers and Cross-Sex Hormones for Minors Outside of Clinical Studies. https://segm.org/Sweden_ends_use_of_Dutch_protocol

Maya Forstater vs CGD and others (2021). Employment Appeal Tribunal. Appeal No. UKEAT/0105/20/JOJ https://assets.publishing.service.gov.uk/media/60c1cce1d3bf7f4bd9814e39/Maya_Forstater_v_CGD_Europe_and_others_UKEAT0105_20_JOJ.pdf

Maya Forstater vs CGD and others (2022). The Employment Tribunal.

Case Number: 2200909/2019. https://www.judiciary.uk/wp-content/uploads/2022/08/Forstater-JR-AG.pdf

BBC. (2021) NHS child gender identity clinic whistleblower wins tribunal. https://www.bbc.co.uk/news/uk-58453250

The Cass Review. (2022). Interim Report. https://cass.independent-review.uk/publications/interim-report/

Cass, H. (2022). Independent review of gender identity services for children and young people - Further advice. https://cass.independent-review.uk/wp-content/uploads/2022/07/Cass-Review-Letter-to-NHSE_19-July-2022.pdf

Hayward, E. (2022). Tavistock gender clinic forced to shut over safety fears - Centre accused of rushing vulnerable children into treatment. The Times. https://www.thetimes.co.uk/article/tavistock-gender-clinic-forced-to-shut-over-safety-fears-wpdx3v6nw

GMC. (2021). Good practice in prescribing and managing medicines and devices. https://www.gmc-uk.org/ethical-guidance/ethical-guidance-for-doctors/good-practice-in-prescribing-and-managing-medicines-and-devices

Hisle-Gorman, E., Schvey, N. A., Adirim, T. A., Rayne, A. K., Susi, A., Roberts, T. A., & Klein, D. A. (2021). Mental Healthcare Utilization of Transgender Youth Before and After Affirming Treatment. The journal of sexual medicine, 18(8), 1444–1454. https://doi.org/10.1016/j.jsxm.2021.05.014

Van Mol, A, Laidlaw, M. K. Grossman, M. McHugh, P. Correction: Transgender Surgery Provides No Mental Health Benefit. https://www.thepublicdiscourse.com/2020/09/71296/

Alzahrani, T. Nguyen, T. Ryan, A. Dwairy, A. McCaffrey, J. Yunus, R. Forgione, J. Krepp, J. Nagy, C. Mazhari, R. Reiner, J. (2019). Cardiovascular Disease Risk Factors and Myocardial Infarction in the Transgender Population. Circulation: Cardiovascular Quality and Outcomes. Vol. 12, No. 4. https://doi.org/10.1161/CIRCOUTCOMES.119.005597

Nota, N. M., Wiepjes, C. M., de Blok, C., Gooren, L., Kreukels, B., & den Heijer, M. (2019). Occurrence of Acute Cardiovascular Events in Transgender Individuals Receiving Hormone Therapy. Circulation, 139(11), 1461–1462. https://doi.org/10.1161/CIRCULATIONAHA.118.038584

RCGP. (2019). The role of the GP in caring for gender-questioning and transgender patients - RCGP Position Statement. https://allcatsrgrey.org.uk/wp/download/management/human_resources/diversity/RCGP-transgender-care-position-statement-june-2019.pdf

@Rebecca35935662. (2022). Are you aware that your Medical School has signed this? On behalf of all students and staff [image of signatures with pronouns next to them]. Twitter. Oct 12, 2022. https://twitter.com/Rebecca35935662/status/1580143117030027264

UK Parliament. (2022). Conversion Therapy (Prohibition) Bill. A Bill to prohibit sexual orientation and gender identity conversion therapy; and for connected purposes. https://bills.parliament.uk/bills/2939

Noll, R. (2013). When Psychiatry Battled the Devil. Psychiatric Times. https://www.researchgate.net/publication/262214055_When_psychiatry_battled_the_devil

Chapter 20

CASE STUDY 4 - BMA Policy Capture

On 16th September 2020, at the annual meeting of British Medical Association (BMA) representatives, which had "diversity" as its theme, the Prioritised Motion 4 brought forward by North West Regional Council asked:

"That this meeting affirms the rights of transgender and nonbinary individuals to access healthcare and live their lives with dignity, including having their identity respected and calls upon the government to:

i) allow transgender and nonbinary individuals to gain legal recognition of their gender by witnessed, sworn statement;

li) ensure that under 18s are able to access healthcare in line with existing principles of consent established by UK Case Law and guidelines published by the public bodies which set the standards for healthcare;

lii) enable trans people to receive healthcare in settings appropriate to their gender identity;

iv) ensure trans healthcare workers are able to access facilities appropriate to the gender they identify as;

v) ensure trans people are able to access gendered spaces in line with the gender they identify;"

Although this Motion seemed rooted in the language of human rights, what it asked for in practice was:

1. De-medicalisation of the process for obtaining a Gender Recognition Certificate by replacing the existing requirements (a gender dysphoria diagnosis, the careful psychological assessment and the proof of living in the "chosen gender role" role for two years), with a sworn statement alone. This would de facto legalise gender self-identification for anyone, including minors.

2. Free access to puberty blockers and cross-sex hormones for children who identify as transgender, based on an informed consent model and WPATH guidelines. This controversial practice was subject to Judicial Review at the time. Three months later, the court found that children could not meaningfully consent to these experimental interventions because the evidence base was lacking, and the treatments could cause sterility and loss of sexual function..

3. Removal of single-sex healthcare facilities and services in favour of mixed-sex ones.

One might think that such an avant-garde policy, based on "choice" and "gender identity" instead of evidence, safeguarding, and biological sex, was a result of prolonged debate and consensus among UK doctors, but that's not what happened.

All the BMA members I know personally, and others who had contacted me in confidence following this meeting, said that the first time they learned about this Motion was shortly before it was put to vote. Despite this, the Chair declined requests for postponement and allowed only 20 minutes for the debate.

During this discussion, which happened online due to Covid

restrictions, the speakers against the Motion were allegedly plagued by sound issues and given less time to speak than their pro-gender self-identification opponents. What resulted could hardly be called a wide-ranging debate, but it was undoubtedly a tense one.

Arguing *for* the Motion, a newly qualified junior doctor and North West Regional Council representative Grace Allport focused on the "rights" and "validity" of trans-identifying people. She claimed that the UK Government, who earlier that year rejected gender self-identification, was threatening to row back transgender rights and deny healthcare to those under 18 who experienced gender dysphoria. She criticised the process for granting Gender Recognition Certificates (GRC) as "costly", "opaque" and all about doctors assessing the "validity" of transition. She said that gender self-identification in countries such as Ireland, Argentina and Norway was "working well".

Dr Angela Dixon, an experienced GP who's been practicing medicine since 1987, argued *against* the motion by drawing attention to medical ethics, evidence-based medicine, and the Equality Act 2010 (EA2010). She said that while it was important for all transgender people to have access to healthcare, the BMA should not be endorsing puberty blockers and hormone treatments for gender dysphoric children, which lack evidence for their usage and could cause irreversible changes to the body, including infertility. She warned that treating "trans women" as women on the basis of gender self-identification impinged on provisions that ensured women could access healthcare safely and with dignity, and asked the BMA not to support legal changes that conflict with women's sex-based rights.

Dr Tom Dolphin, a BMA Council member, equated resistance to gender self-identification to Section 28, claiming that just like gay people thirty years ago, trans-identifying people were "victims of a culture war" and "subject to moral panic". (Trueland, 2020)

Eventually, out of 159,000 BMA members and 250 delegates who were present at this meeting, only 125 delegates voted. The result was split 49% for the motion and 36% against, with a substantial number abstaining from voting.

Following the vote, a colleague sent me a side by side comparison of two briefs.

Version 1 dates back to October 2018, when the BMA Medical Ethics Committee met to consider the issue of gender self-identification, in relation to the Government's consultation on amendments to the Gender Recognition Act. After a lengthy debate, no firm conclusion was reached about whether the BMA should support a simplified process for the legal recognition of transgender individuals. Without a clear position on the key questions, the BMA did not respond to that consultation.

VERSION 1	VERSION 2
(Cisgender) The terms for those whose gender identity is the same as their sex. It is often abbreviated to 'cis'.	(Cisgender) The term for those whose gender identity is the same as their sex assigned at birth. It is often abbreviated to 'cis'.
Given the emphasis elsewhere in medical law and ethics on the autonomous choices of competent adult patients, it has been suggested that a requirement for medical involvement in a process that has widely been argued to be 'non-medical' may be unsustainable; *if it is accepted that individuals know their own gender, then medical involvement in determining it may be superfluous**	Given the emphasis elsewhere in medical law and ethics on the autonomous choices of competent adult patients, it has been suggested that a requirement for medical involvement in a process that has widely been argued to be 'non-medical' may be unsustainable.
Concerns have also been raised that expediting the process of legal recognition could have unintended effects on historically single-sex spaces. There have been a small number of high-profile cases where the process of self-identification has been used by those in detention settings to gain access to single sex spaces in order to commit abuses. While these cases are both numerically and proportionally very small, they are demonstrative of the potential for manipulation in environments where individuals are already in a vulnerable situation. Concern has been expressed that a simplified process could increase this risk. Conversely, though, it is argued that trans people being forced into environments which do not align with their gender identity puts them at risk of abuse and violence.	REMOVED
Patients receiving healthcare are often in a vulnerable position and every reasonable effort should be made to ensure they are as comfortable as possible. This includes trans people. It should also be noted that cis people should receive healthcare in appropriate settings and having trans people in that environment may not necessarily be suitable. It is argued, however, that this does not preclude trans people from receiving healthcare in settings appropriate to their gender identity, as suitable adjustments can be made. For example, trans women will still have a prostate gland and need to receive suitable treatment in relation to this.	Patients receiving healthcare are often in a vulnerable position and every reasonable effort should be made to ensure they are as comfortable as possible. This includes trans people and cis people. Some cis people have argued that in certain healthcare environments, cis people and trans people should be separate. It is argued, however, that this does not preclude trans people from receiving healthcare in settings appropriate to their gender identity, as suitable adjustments can be made. For example, trans women will still have a prostate gland and may need to receive suitable treatment in relation to this, which may include being treated on a women's ward.

VERSION 1	VERSION 2
This part of the motion also focuses on the rights and wishes of trans people being respected, though there is a potential tension with the sensibilities of cis people. This is covered in depth in the briefings for part (iii) and part (v).	This part of the motion also focuses on the rights and wishes of trans people being upheld. As highlighted in other parts of the briefing ((iii) and (v)) there is a potential tension with the sensibilities of some cis people.
Others see the issue differently. While the rights of trans people should be respected, it is argued that the rights of cis people need to be recognised in this context also. There may be legitimate concerns about cis people sharing certain spaces with trans people, especially when they are in a vulnerable position. This has been a particular concern with regard to support services for cis women who have been exposed to severely traumatic and abusive experiences at the hands of men; it may be necessary for them to be able to seek spaces restricted to cis women in order to feel sufficiently safe and secure to access the support and help they need.	REMOVED
If restrictions on access to gendered spaces exist, how they are enforced and what impact this could have on individuals who do not conform to stereotypical gender norms should also be considered.	The BMA is aware of other points of view on this issue, including that some cis people have raised concerns about sharing certain spaces with trans people.

After the vote, doctors who supported Motion 4 took to Twitter to celebrate.

Dr Dolphin expressed satisfaction that the Motion had passed in full and warned "transphobes" that should they "pile on" he would "mute" them. (@thomasdolphin, 2020 (1); @thomasdolphin, 2020 (2))

By "transphobes" and "piling on" Dr Dolphin seemed to be referring to numerous polite questions, and expressions of concern about gender self-identification, from members of the public as well as other doctors.

A newly qualified junior doctor Emma Runswick was also delighted that the Motion she had worked so hard on had passed, and said she welcomed questions about it.

A Twitter user whose daughter has learning disabilities

replied, asking Dr Runswick how she would guarantee her daughter's boundaries weren't breached when she ends up hospitalised and placed in a bed next to a male patient. (@Dis_Critic, 2020)

Dr Runswick replied that safeguarding polices apply regardless of "gender", that hospitals have single-en-suite rooms and that "trans women" weren't any more of a threat to her daughter than "cis women". (@ERunswickBMA, 2020 (1))

What followed was many Twitter users presenting evidence to the contrary. Men who identify as women are well-known to retain male-pattern criminality (Dhejne, 2011). Ministry of Justice figures show that over half of transgender inmates in UK prisons are sex offenders (Fair Play For Women, 2017). When these men are admitted onto female-only wards, female patients who raise concerns are gaslit and accused of "bigotry" by NHS staff (Helyar et al, 2021).

Instead of taking a moment to reflect on this new evidence, Dr Runswick described it as a "pile on" and claimed that her detractors didn't understand UK law. (@ERunswickBMA, 2020 (2); @ERunswickBMA (3))

This is a common transactivist response, which stems from the confusion about the way the GRA2004 and the EA2010 interact with each other in practice.

The GRA2004 states that once full GRC has been granted, "the person's gender becomes for all purposes the acquired gender (so that, if the acquired gender is the male gender, the person's sex becomes that of a man and, if it is the female gender, the person's sex becomes that of a woman)" (Gender Recognition Act, 2004).

This disregards the immutable nature of biological sex, on which women's sex-based rights hinge.

The EA2010 attempted to address this discrepancy by

differentiating between the protected characteristics of "sex" and "gender reassignment".

The Act defined "woman" as a "female of any age" and "man" as a "male of any age". These two groups - which encompass every person in the UK - have the protected characteristic of "sex".

"Transsexual" is defined as a person who has undergone, or is proposing to undergo, gender reassignment by changing physiological or other attributes of their sex. These individuals share the protected characteristic of "gender reassignment".

Section 29 of the EA2010 states that those who provide a service to the public must not discriminate against persons who require that service.

However, in Part 7, the Act specifies that Section 29 is not contravened by providing single-sex services in situations where a joint service for both sexes would be less effective and where single-sex service is *a proportionate means of achieving a legitimate aim*.

Assessing this "on case by case basis" doesn't mean that each individual male should be risk assessed by frontline staff, in order to decide whether he should be included or excluded from a female-only service. It refers to assessing the *type* of service that is provided. If it can be shown that the service itself is a proportionate means of achieving a legitimate aim - for example a rape crisis service or a hospital ward being female-only in order to provide safety and dignity to female service users - then all males, regardless of whether they have a GRC and/or a self-declared gender identity, can be excluded from it as a matter of policy.

In the Explanatory notes, the Act gives examples of situations where single-sex exemptions are permitted. Unsurprisingly, one of the most common areas is healthcare, especially with regards to single-sex facilities such as hospital wards and bathrooms, single-sex services such as maternity and health screening, and access to same-sex healthcare providers (Equality Act, 2010).

Unfortunately, both GRA2004 and EA2010 have been systematically misrepresented to justify prioritising gender self-identification over biological sex. This has resulted in the *de facto* disappearance of women's single-sex spaces and provisions.

Reflecting on what happened at the BMA conference, I was reminded of *Only adults? Good practices in legal gender recognition for youth - A report on the current state of laws and NGO advocacy in eight countries in Europe, with a focus on rights of young people* (Dentons, IGLYO, et al, 2019).

The strategies outlined in this document include:

1. Target youth politicians. Because main wings of political parties are usually keen to listen to the younger generation, and youth politicians of today are senior politicians of the future, any changes to policies they are in favour of are supposedly more likely to be "on the right side of history".

2. De-medicalise the campaign. In most countries, legally changing gender involves obtaining a diagnosis of gender dysphoria and undergoing some degree of social or medical gender reassignment. As one of the main criticisms of allowing minors to change their gender has involved opposition to irreversible medical treatments before the age of maturity, it is suggested that resistance would lessen if activists educated the public that legal gender change was a purely administrative process..

3. Get ahead of the government agenda and the media story. This could be achieved by publishing progressive legislative proposals before the government has a chance to develop its own. The document warns that failing to intervene early could cause the eventual gender recognition legislation to be less progressive than activists would like it to be.

4. Use human rights as a campaign point to highlight human rights of trans-identifying people. People who sought to legally change gender in Norway apparently had to undergo sterilisation procedures (although this requirement did not appear in formal legislation). Activists rightfully argued that this breached trans-identifying people's human rights, which helped them to legalise gender self-identification.

5. Tie your campaign to a more popular reform. This worked equally well in Denmark, Norway and Ireland, where "marriage equality was strongly supported, but gender identity remained a more difficult issue to win public support for".

6. Avoid excessive press coverage and exposure. In countries such as the UK, the opposition to changes in gender recognition law was seen to arise because "information on legal gender recognition reforms has been misinterpreted in the mainstream media". Therefore the report suggests that directly lobbying individual politicians and keeping press coverage to a minimum, as well as developing strong ties with youth politicians who can present the changes to gender recognition laws to the senior members of their parties, could have more success.

7. Carpe diem. Activists are advised to "seize the moment" and "quickly capitalise on political momentum" when promoting gender self-identification.

I don't know the demographics of most BMA representatives who were present at the meeting, but the representatives who promoted Motion 4 on social media all appeared young and political.

They argued for the de-medicalisation of gender recognition, encouraged the BMA to get ahead of the government on trans rights and claimed there was "overwhelming support" for gender self-identification, even though official data do not support this assertion. (Fair Play for Women, 2018; Campbell, 2020)

Motion 4 was selectively framed in terms of the human rights of trans and non-binary people, while the evidence of the possible negative impact on the human rights of women was removed from the brief.

The Motion was also tied to the more popular cause of "diversity and inclusiveness", with delegates who argued for the Motion likening gender self-identification to gay rights.

Excessive exposure and coverage was certainly avoided by ensuring most delegates only became aware of the Motion shortly before it was put to vote, while "carpe diem" was enacted by denying requests for extension, allocating only 20 minutes to the debate and pushing the Motion through on the same day.

There's another strategy outlined in the Denton's report - **Use case studies of real people** - which advises activists to tell human interest stories in order to increase empathy and support for their cause.

This is indeed what many women did in response to the announcement that the BMA had endorsed gender self-identification.

I offered to speak to the BMA about this policy's impact on women (@lascapigliata8, 2020).

Several Twitter users shared experiences of sexual assault in healthcare settings. They pointed out that disabled women were at increased risk of abuse, which is why access to same-sex intimate care providers and facilities was essential for their health and well-being.

Others shared news stories that evidenced the abuse women experienced as a consequence of mixed-sex hospital wards and gender self-identification policies.

In Ireland, where gender self-identification is legal, a 17 year old girl was raped by men in a hospital room (Michael, 2020).

In the UK, a female patient who was sectioned during a manic episode was labelled "transphobic" by staff when she complained about the presence of a trans-identified male patient on the women's ward (Lancaster Guardian, 2018).

Also in the UK, a man who identified as a woman was found to be using public Wi-Fi to access child abuse content from his hospital bed (Gordon, 2020).

The BMA members complained to the BMA directly about how Motion 4 was handled, and some even cancelled their BMA memberships in protest.

Bev Jackson of LGB Alliance UK, who campaigns for the rights of gay, lesbian and bisexual people, warned the BMA against "denying biological reality" and becoming a "laughing stock" (Ridler, 2020).

None of this made a difference. The BMA did not engage with us on Twitter and later on, in response to a letter in the BMJ, they denied that by endorsing gender self-identification, the BMA effectively supported changing women's single-sex spaces into mixed-sex (Chisholm, 2021).

Eventually, the conversation on social media and in clinician groups turned to the deeply entrenched sexism within the BMA, which was exposed in a series of news articles in 2019 after female doctors spoke out about being belittled and harassed by the BMA officials, including having their thighs and buttocks fondled, being propositioned after a policy speech, and male colleagues sending them naked photos and trying to guess their bra size (Smyth, 2019).

Subsequent investigation found "a 'toxic' atmosphere for women", and described the BMA as an "old boys' club, in which female staff are regularly demeaned, patronised and sexually harassed".

The BMA officials described these findings as "appalling" and vowed to introduce an "external 'guardian of safe working' and internal 'staff listening champions'" (Burgess, 2019).

Considering the circumstances in which the BMA endorsed gender self-identification, I am sorry to say that whatever they did to address institutional sexism in their organisation was nowhere near enough.

Bibliography

Trueland, J. (2020). Push for progress on transgender rights in healthcare. The BMA. https://www.bma.org.uk/news-and-opinion/push-for-progress-on-transgender-rights-in-healthcare

@thomasdolphin. (2020 (1)). @TheBMA #ARM2020 is debating trans rights. I spoke in favour of Motion 4 because trans people need the support of doctors and the BMA, particularly at a time they are the focus of a moral panic - pleased that it has passed in full. [image of Prioritised Motion 4]. Twitter. 16 Sep, 2020. https://twitter.com/thomasdolphin/status/1305835113461231618

@thomasdolphin. (2020 (2)). For the transphobes joining this thread, please save your energy. The BMA is not your enemy and piling on will just result in muting. Twitter. 16 Sep, 2020. https://twitter.com/thomasdolphin/status/1305971453058260996

@DIS_Critic. (2020). My daughter has learning difficulties. She's likely to be hospitalised at points through her adult life. She'll be a vulnerable patient. How will you guarantee her boundaries are not breached? How will you ensure her dignity remains intact if a male patient is in the next bed? Twitter. 16 Sep, 2020. https://twitter.com/Dis_Critic/status/1306244791831797761

@ERunswickBMA. (2020 (1)). Hey - we have existing safeguarding policies for all people, that would apply regardless of the gender of her neighbour. Some hospitals, especially mental health hospitals, have single and en-suite rooms. Trans women are not more of a threat to your daughter than cis women. Twitter. 16 Sep, 2020. https://twitter.com/ERunswickBMA/status/1306320685644615680

Dhejne, C. Lichtenstein, P. Boman, M. Johansson, A.L.V. Långström, N. et al. (2011). Long-Term Follow-Up of Transsexual Persons Undergoing Sex Reassignment Surgery: Cohort Study in Sweden. PLOS ONE 6(2): e16885. https://doi.org/10.1371/journal.pone.0016885

Fair Play for Women (2017). Half of all transgender prisoners are sex offenders or dangerous category A inmates. Fair Play For Women. https://fairplayforwomen.com/transgender-prisoners/

Helyar, S. Hill, A. Griffin, L. (2021). Nurses request that health and nursing organisations withdraw from Stonewall's Diversity Championship Scheme.

https://lascapigliata.com/institutional-capture/nurses-request-that-health-and-nursing-organisations-withdraw-from-stonewalls-diversity-championship-scheme/

@ERunswickBMA. (2020 (2)). I've done my best to respond to the good faith questions in the pile on today. I'm #proud of the stand @THEBMA has made for trans rights and the part I played. #TransRights #BWithTheT. Twitter. 16 Sep, 2020. https://twitter.com/ERunswickBMA/status/1306344639834750976

@ERunswickBMA. (2020 (3)) What has shocked me: -so-called feminists who think a mid-20s qualified Dr is too young/naive to have an opinion -how phallocentric their definition of lesbianism is (women loving women is a positive thing people!) -widespread misunderstanding of current law and practice. 16 Sep, 2020. https://twitter.com/ERunswickBMA/status/1306344658734329856

Gender Recognition Act. (2004). https://www.legislation.gov.uk/ukpga/2004/7/section/9

Equality Act 2010. "212(1) General Interpretation". https://www.legislation.gov.uk/ukpga/2010/15/section/212?wrap=true&view=plain ; Protected characteristic: Sex. https://www.legislation.gov.uk/ukpga/2010/15/section/11 ; Protected characteristic: Gender reassignment. https://www.legislation.gov.uk/ukpga/2010/15/section/7 ; Part 7: Separate, single and concessionary services. https://www.legislation.gov.uk/ukpga/2010/15/schedule/3/part/7 ; Part 7: Separate and single sex services. Separate services for the sexes: Paragraph 26. https://www.legislation.gov.uk/ukpga/2010/15/notes/division/3/16/20/7

Dentons, IGLYO, Thomas Reuters Foundation (2019). Only adults? Good practices in legal gender recognition for youth - A report on the current state of laws and NGO advocacy in eight countries in Europe, with a focus on rights of young people. https://www.iglyo.com/wp-content/uploads/2019/11/IGLYO_v3-1.pdf

Fair Play for Women. (2018). The results of the Populus on-line survey following the UK Gender Recognition Act consultation 2018. https://fairplayforwomen.com/poll/

Campbell, S. (2020). Transforming the question. Wings Over Scotland. Available at: https://wingsoverscotland.com/transforming-the-question/

@lascapigliata8. (2020). Because it appears neither @TheBMA or the @gmcuk have done ANY impact assessment before they declared support for gender self-ID, here's the offer - as a rape survivor and a doctor I'm willing to talk to you about impact these policies are having on women. Any takers? Twitter. 16 Sep, 2020. https://twitter.com/lascapigliata8/status/1306250496072732674

Michael, N. (2020). Campaigners call for Cork University Hospital to end 'shocking silence' over assault. Irish Examiner. https://www.irishexaminer.com/news/arid-30985999.html

Lancaster Guardian. (2018). Lancaster mum with 'fear of men' locked on hospital ward with transgender patient. https://www.lancasterguardian.co.uk/news/lancaster-mum-fear-men-locked-hospital-ward-transgender-patient-653048

Gordon, A. (2020). Trans woman, 54, who used public Wi-Fi to access child porn from hospital bed is jailed for nine months after police find hoard of 80,000 images on laptop - as authorities decide whether to send her to male or female prison. Mail Online. https://www.dailymail.co.uk/news/article-8521787/Paedophile-54-used-public-Wi-Fi-download-child-porn-hospital.html

Ridler, F. (2020). Critics blast BMA for treating 'any man with a beard and penis as a woman' as long as they they identify as female - after it said transgender people should not need a doctor's consent to change gender. Mail Online. https://www.dailymail.co.uk/news/article-8738269/Transgender-people-allowed-change-gender-without-doctors-consent-UK.html?fbclid=IwAR22cxsSKS6go9tuWUhCYEu4MdVnVGzD1pI1IyfS-VRg6MCoCozZ3Uhshss

Chisholm, J. (2021). BMA response to Dr Bowen, Dr Clyde, Dr Wright et al. The BMJ. https://www.bmj.com/content/372/bmj.n205/rapid-responses

Smyth, C. (2019). GPs quit union amid anger at 70s-style sexism. The Times. https://www.thetimes.co.uk/article/gps-quit-union-amid-anger-at-70s-style-sexism-pfw2pjvsr

Burgess, K. (2019). BMA accused of calling its women doctors 'silly girls'. The Times. https://www.thetimes.co.uk/article/bma-accused-of-calling-its-women-doctors-silly-girls-jhlldwtgz

Chapter 21

Examples of Gender Ideology in Medical Institutions

For over a decade, UK medical institutions were given erroneous interpretations of the Equality Act (EA2010), specifically relating to the protected characteristics of "sex" and "gender reassignment".

The errors typically included:

1. Replacing the protected characteristic of "sex" with "gender".

Sex is clearly defined in UK law. "Woman" means "a female of any age" and "man" means "a male of any age". The definitions of "male", "female", "man" and "woman" in all human languages are sex-based. Male and female bodies differ anatomically and physiologically, which has clinical implications.

On the other hand, "gender" isn't clearly defined. Originating as a linguistic term, "gender" is used to denote the sex-role stereotypes of masculinity and femininity, which are in a large part socially constructed. "Gender" has subsequently evolved into a polite euphemism for biological sex, although this has never been formalised in law or science.

Prior to the emergence of gender ideology, it was understood that phrases such as "gender-based violence" or "gender pay-gap" referred to male violence against women and the pay gap between the two sexes, respectively.

When the word "gender" appeared in medical literature, we could be confident that it referred to biological sex.

Now, thanks to years of aggressive campaigning to conflate sex and gender in language, policy and law, and to permit men and women to self-identify as the opposite sex, both patients and healthcare staff who identify as "trans" are being mis-sexed in clinical settings. This has compromised data collection, patient welfare and equality monitoring.

2. Replacing the protected characteristic of "gender reassignment" with "gender identity".

According to the EA2010, anyone who has transitioned, or is proposing to transition to the opposite sex-role (gender), has a protected characteristic of "gender reassignment". This holds true regardless of whether these individuals have Gender Recognition Certificates (GRCs) or not.

Obtaining a GRC involves getting a diagnosis of Gender Identity Disorder (now replaced with Gender Dysphoria), careful medical assessment, and living in the opposite sex-role for two years. As a consequence, only a few thousand people in the UK have GRCs.

Contrary to common belief, genital surgery was never a requirement for obtaining a GRC, and evidence shows that the vast majority of men who identify as women retain their natural genitals (Nolan et al, 2019).

Although the goal of granting GRCs was not to erase sex in language, law or medicine, it has set the precedent of legally aiding individuals to falsify sex markers on their documents, including birth certificates.

Since the advent of gender ideology, the concept of "gender identity" as an "internal sense of being male or female" has emerged. This has strengthened some people's belief that individuals who identify as the opposite sex "must have been born in the wrong body", that gender identity - not our biological sex - determines whether we are male or female, and that GRCs are either superfluous or that they should be issued based on self-declaration rather than as a part of a regulated process which involves medical gatekeeping.

By replacing the protected characteristic of "gender reassignment" with "gender identity" (which is neither a protected characteristic under the EA2010 nor a scientifically valid concept), gender ideology pressure groups have managed to convince authorities to embed gender self-identification practices not only in healthcare settings, but in all other walks of life. Now that males are allowed to self-identify as females, and females as males, anyone can request a change of their sex marker on documents such as drivers licences, passports, NHS and even prison records. To refuse to go along with this attracts accusations of "discrimination", "hate crime" and "transphobia".

3. Promoting the law as Stonewall UK wants it to be.

In 2015, LGB organisation Stonewall UK rebranded itself as LGBT to include activism for trans rights in their remit. Ever since, LGBT+ organisations have been campaigning for gender self-identification, paediatric gender reassignment and the removal of single-sex exemptions from the EA2010. (Stonewall, 2015; Stonewall 2020)

As a result, every institution in the UK that had an ongoing relationship with Stonewall from the days when Stonewall championed the rights of LGB people automatically signed up to champion these new goals. This was facilitated through various Stonewall schemes, such as the Workplace Equality Index and the Stonewall Champions list.

Once the scandal of Stonewall's influence on UK institutions broke out and organisations started leaving, Stonewall removed the list of Stonewall Champions from their website (Sex Matters, 2021). However, in its heyday, all major UK institutions and most big businesses were among the 800-odd members, and they used their influence to promote Stonewall's campaign as if it was the law.

As far as I know, the General Medical Council (GMC), Nursing and Midwifery Council (NMC), most NHS Trusts, medical and nursing schools, hospitals, and Royal Colleges are still either Stonewall Champions or fully signed up to one of Stonewall's schemes. Consequently, women's single-sex spaces have disappeared from healthcare settings without a word of opposition from the elite medical leadership. This happened even though humans can't change sex, there is no evidence of a biological basis for gender identity, and the law clearly distinguishes between sex and gender.

I must admit I still struggle to understand how anyone - medically qualified or not - can pretend not to know that a woman is an adult human female, let alone how they can watch women being discriminated against, and endangered, in their most vulnerable moments. It is also unacceptable that many are condemning the women who are complaining about their human rights being trampled on. I will however, resist the urge to speculate on the reasons behind otherwise responsible adults allowing this travesty to pass. Instead, I would like to move on to concrete examples of the ideological capture of medical institutions by gender ideology, and following that, to some real-life examples of how this is affecting the practice of medicine, medical education and patient welfare.

General Medical Council (GMC)

Patients can no longer depend on the medical regulator in the UK to truthfully record a clinician's biological sex, because the GMC allows doctors to self-identify as male or female. The process to change one's sex marker is described in the 'Maintain your registration' section of the GMC website, under the heading 'Changing your name and gender status'. To change their name, a doctor needs to fill out an application form and provide documentary evidence of their old name and a new name. The GMC suggests that this can be a passport, but if a doctor doesn't have this, they are willing to accept "alternative evidence".

The GMC does not require any evidence of a change in gender status; the request is enough.

Once the application is received, the GMC says it will issue two separate GMC records for the same doctor - one in their old name and with the old sex marker, and the other in their new name and with the new sex marker. The two records will have a different GMC number and there will be no link between them (GMC, no date (1)).

On the 'Ethical hub - Trans healthcare' section of the GMC website, under a tab 'Confidentiality and equality', the GMC advises that doctors should also change their patient's sex marker upon request, and likewise, no evidence of change in a patient's gender status - such as a Gender Recognition Certificate - is required (GMC, no date (2)).

Once the sex marker is changed - a procedure that is facilitated by Primary Care Support England (PCSE) - the patient is issued with a new NHS number, and has to re-register with their practice as a new patient. As all evidence of their biological sex is removed from the new record, it is up to the doctor to discuss repercussions with the patient, including the fact that they will no longer be automatically invited for sex-appropriate health screening (PCSE, no date; LGBT Foundation, 2020).

According to the GMC, "gender status or history of trans-identified and non-binary patients should be treated with the same degree of confidentiality as any other sensitive personal information", and doctors are advised that it is "unlawful to disclose a patient's gender history without their consent". Previously, I could not find any relevant caveats to this recommendation. However, when I checked the GMC website in November 2022, I saw that they made an exception for disclosures to other healthcare professionals for the purpose of preventative medicine, diagnosis and provision of care and treatment, as well as if the clinician who is making a disclosure reasonably believes that the subject has given consent, or cannot give such consent (GMC, no date (2). This is a welcome clarification indeed. However, in a video titled 'How to make your practice more inclusive' the GMC claims that "not everything's about gender" and they use a clinical scenario of a patient presenting with a broken elbow as an example where "gender identity just isn't relevant" (GMC, no date (3)).

Just to be clear: knowingly changing a patient's sex-marker to the opposite sex constitutes deliberate mis-sexing, because biological sex is immutable. A male doesn't stop being male just because some of his documents have been changed to "female", and vice versa. Therefore, apart from the inherent absurdity of the medical regulator advising doctors to mis-sex patients, suggesting that the patient's biological sex would be irrelevant in any clinical scenario is incorrect and also unsafe.

For example, it is very important to ascertain the biological sex of a patient who needs an X-ray for a broken arm, because if they are female they could be pregnant. As for gender identity and the past medical history of gender reassignment, a previous use of puberty blockers and cross-sex hormones is known to result in bone thinning, which is why it too is relevant.

Furthermore, whether or not gender self-identification is legal in the UK, it cannot be "unlawful" for a doctor to pass on essential information such as the patient's biological sex to other healthcare professionals, with or without the patient's consent.

On their pages, the GMC uses a scenario in which a trans-identified male patient reports being upset that the receptionist at the GP practice was confused when a man's voice on the phone claimed to be "Angela".

However, a far more relevant example would be one of, say, a female patient who identifies as a man and who is in a relationship with a male who identifies as a woman, presenting with a suspected ectopic pregnancy. Or an unconscious trauma victim, who happens to be a man dressed in women's clothing with a drivers' licence showing a female name and a female sex marker.

If a doctor cannot obtain consent from a female patient to order a pregnancy test - perhaps because she is adamant that "as a man who is in a relationship with a woman he cannot possibly be pregnant" - or if the doctor can't obtain consent from an unconscious patient to indicate on a blood form that he is indeed male, would the GMC really want the doctor to proceed treating these acutely unwell patients as if they were in fact the opposite sex? What happens if a patient suffers serious injury or even dies as a consequence of being mis-sexed in a medical emergency? Who will be held legally and morally responsible?

I would prefer to be reassured that the GMC would have my back should a patient, who had survived thanks to my sex-appropriate diagnosis and treatment, decide to lodge a complaint about "misgendering". Unfortunately, judging by the GMC advice at the time of writing of this essay, no doctor can be sure of that.

The impact of this goes beyond individual doctors and patients.

Doctors who are working in prisons, for example, are being compelled to change sex markers on the medical records of male sex offenders. This can affect risk assessment as well as be used to initiate the transfer of these men to the female estate and their placement on female medical wards, both of which endanger women.

Gender self-identification policies also compel clinicians to gaslight and even abuse female patients.

In 2018, a Lancaster mum whose bi-polar disorder left her believing men were conspiring to kill her was locked on a women's psychiatric ward with a man who identified as a woman. Despite her being terrified of this man, her concerns were not taken seriously and she was labelled a "transphobic bigot" by the staff (Lancaster Guardian, 2018).

In 2022, Baroness Emma Nicholson revealed in the House of Lords that a woman had been raped in hospital by a trans-identified man. However, when the woman reported the assault to the police, the hospital claimed that she could not have been raped as there were no male patients on the ward. It took a year, CCTV footage and witnesses coming forward, before the hospital finally admitted that there was man on the women's ward after all, and that the rape had occurred. (Beal, 2022).

British Medical Association (BMA)

In 2020, the BMA passed the Prioritised Motion 4, asking the BMA to support a) gender self-identification for both patients and clinicians, b) full access to spaces and facilities "appropriate to the gender they identify as" and c) consent-based access to paediatric gender reassignment for under 18s (Trueland, 2020).

After the BMA endorsed this motion, the High Court paused the prescription of puberty blockers for gender dysphoria, citing concerns about the poor evidence-base and disputing that children as young as 10 are Gillick competent to consent to future sterility and loss of sexual function. These irreversible side-effects typically result from puberty blocker treatment progressing to cross sex hormones, which happens in 98% of puberty blocked gender dysphoric minors according to the Tavistock's own study (Carmichael et al, 2021).

Many doctors in the UK who had been concerned about the harms of paediatric gender reassignment for some time breathed a sigh of relief. However, Tavistock GIDS announced that they would be appealing the decision, and the BMA was reported to be considering whether or not to intervene on Tavistock's behalf.

In an exchange via Rapid Responses to the BMJ article 'Gender dysphoria service rated inadequate after waiting list of 4600 raises concerns', a group of doctors questioned the ethics of such a BMA intervention. They also expressed concerns about the process by which Motion 4 was endorsed at the BMA conference and pointed out that the BMA advocating for gender self-identification in healthcare settings effectively changes women's single-sex spaces into mixed-sex. (Bowen et al, 2021)

In reply to their concerns, the Head of the BMA Medical Ethics Committee Dr John Chisholm, cited the Gillick competence argument and rebuffed concerns regarding Motion 4 by claiming that the "BMA's policy was made through our well-established democratic process". He added that "it is also important to be clear that the BMA has not (as the authors suggest) sought to change 'women's single-sex spaces into mixed-sex'" (Chisholm, 2021).

In support of his assertion, Dr Chisholm linked to the BMA response to the UK government's 'Women and Equalities Committee Inquiry on Reform of the Gender Recognition Act' where the BMA had advocated for change of legal gender to require nothing more than a sworn statement. In the section on single-sex and separate sex services and facilities, the BMA claimed that "some cis people have argued that in certain healthcare environments cis people and trans people should be separate. It is argued, however, that this does not preclude trans people from receiving healthcare in settings appropriate to their gender identity, as suitable adjustments can be made. It has been suggested that these issues could be resolved by ensuring the appropriate privacy, dignity and confidentiality of all patients. Further guidance should clearly aim to remove discrimination and support all people to safe use of services" (BMA, 2020).

It is interesting that the BMA chose to misrepresent separate services for males and females as separate services for "cis people and trans people". The whole point of single-sex provisions is that trans-identifying patients would be accommodated on the wards consistent with their biological sex, which means they would be accommodated *alongside* people of the same sex who are not trans-identifying (or in BMA parlance, trans people would be accommodated with cis people of the same sex). More worryingly, the blanket statement that people who don't identify as the opposite sex are necessarily "cis" betrays the fact that the BMA seems to think that most women identify with oppressive gender stereotypes of femininity.

Be that as it may, the BMA offers no practical solutions for how they would ensure the appropriate privacy, dignity, and confidentiality for everyone in hospitals where there are only mixed-sex wards thanks to gender self-identification policies, and side rooms are both scarce and not always the best place for sick patients. Their recommendations seem myopically focused on pushing gender self-identification, and they don't meaningfully acknowledge the impact of that on other protected groups, such as women, the disabled, the elderly and religious groups, for whom same-sex care and facilities are paramount.

At the last check, before Stonewall removed the list of its champions from public view, the BMA were a member of their Diversity Champion scheme.

Care Quality Commission (CQC)

Discussing why they replaced "sex" (protected characteristic) with "gender" (not a protected characteristic) in their Equality policy, the CQC tweeted:

"There's nothing in Act that says that we need to use a specific word for a protected characteristic. When we use gender as a descriptor of one of the protected characteristics (as we do in equality monitoring form), there's no evidence to show that we are excluding anyone (2/3)" (@CareQualityComm, 2020).

In 2016 and 2017, when the CQC inspected a GP surgery that employs a male GP who identifies as a woman, they did not note any concerns regarding the impact this could have on female patients. They only referred to patients being treated by clinicians of the same "gender" and the word "sex" does not appear in their report (Forstater, 2020; CQC, 2016; CQC, 2017).

This is despite CQC's own investigation into sexual assaults on mental health wards, which revealed a very bleak picture for women patients, and highlighted how crucial is to collect data based on sex (CQC, 2018).

Medical education

In the UK, apart from the teaching hospitals and universities being Stonewall Diversity Champions, medical schools are also members of the Athena SWAN award scheme. This appears to be organised through the Medical Schools Council (MCS), a representative body that consists of the heads of every UK medical school, who meet in order to shape medical education in the UK.

On their Athena SWAN page, the MCS states:

"In 2011, the Chief Medical Officer announced that the National Institute for Health Research would only accept medical schools which have attained a 'silver' Athena SWAN award to be shortlisted for research funding. This acted as a powerful motivator for engagement with Athena SWAN. While a silver award is no longer a criteria for NIHR funding, the Athena SWAN Charter remains an unrivalled evidence base for NIHR applicants to demonstrate commitment to equality, diversity and inclusion. The MSC provides a source of assistance for medical schools that are seeking to apply for Athena SWAN awards" (Medical Schools Council, 2021).

Athena SWAN originally set out to address the inequality of women in STEM, and despite the fact that they, too, are using "gender" as a more polite euphemism for "biological sex", their pages mainly talk about equality for "females". They also correctly include "sex" and "gender reassignment" on their lists of protected characteristics.

However, once you look at Athena SWAN's definition of "intersectionality", "sex" is replaced by "gender".

Digging deeper into the Athena SWAN guidance, it quickly becomes apparent that "sex" is now subsumed and entirely overruled by "gender" and that Athena SWAN's goals have changed.

For example, their Gender Equality Guidance starts off by defining terms such as "gender roles", "gender identity" and "gender expression" and it goes on to say, "These different aspects of gender have typically been understood as binary: male and female, men and women. However, gender does not represent a simple binary choice, it is more fluid. A person's gender is self-determined by their internal perception, identification and experience. Therefore, a person's gender identity may not be the same as the sex the individual was registered as at birth. It may also change over time" (Advance HE, 2020).

Being female doesn't "change over time". It is a fundamental sex-based axis of oppression all women and girls have to contend with and it is these primary inequalities that Athena SWAN was designed to mitigate. Unfortunately, Athena SWAN now advocates for "gender disaggregated data" and makes no distinction between women and the men who self-identify as women. This compromises sex-disaggregated data which are needed to highlight sex-based discrimination.

This document also doesn't link to any resources that are designed to address the sex-based inequalities women suffer. Instead they link to another Advance HE page which is filled with trans-focused guidance and resources.

One of the documents on this page is *Trans staff and students in HE and colleges: improving experiences*. It starts off with a gender ideology-influenced glossary of terms, and while it clearly devotes a lot of attention to both the legal and practical aspects of helping trans-identifying people, it also promotes gender self-identification for students and staff. By advising universities that trans people should be allowed to use single-sex facilities in line with "self-identified gender" it also compromises single-sex provisions under the EA2010. It, additionally, recommends that institutions should have a trans equality policy (Pugh, 2016).

This "Trans equality policy statement" is designed to be copy/pasted by institutions, as it provides space for (institution name) throughout. The transactivist rhetoric is significantly ramped up in this document, which at one point defines "unwanted questions" directed at trans-identified people as "transphobic abuse" and it vows to promptly remove any "transphobic propaganda" - including written material and speeches - from campus (Equality Challenge Unit, 2016).

Let's consider an obvious example that I know has played out many times. These documents instruct universities (including medical schools) to allow men who self-identify as women to use female toilets. If a woman was to find herself in a toilet with such a man, she might ask him what he was doing there, which could be construed as an "unwanted question" and labelled as "transphobic abuse" - not just by the boundary transgressing man but by the university itself. If this woman tried to explain why she wasn't comfortable with a man in female toilets - or heaven forbid if she wrote something in order to raise awareness of how gender self-identification is impacting on women's sex-based rights - she could be accused of spreading "transphobic propaganda". This would make it a lot easier to target her with disciplinary procedures, which could in turn threaten her place at the university.

Now imagine a female patient requests a female clinician in a teaching hospital that is signed up to the Athena SWAN scheme, and instead of a woman, a trans-identified man turns up.

Since I've been involved in feminist activism, I have read many distressing testimonies from women about the way their requests for female-only nursing care are being disregarded by the health services.

In one such case, a woman had requested female-only nursing care following a colonoscopy, because she also suffered from urge incontinence and knew she would need intimate care after the procedure. She confided in her GP about the reasons why she found colonoscopy particularly challenging, and was reassured that she would have access to female-only intimate care. However, when she woke up from the anaesthetic, she was shocked to find a trans-identified male nurse pinning her down.

Although she said she thought of nothing else afterwards, she was reluctant to complain because she didn't trust that the hospital would not treat her as the problem, and as a chronic illness patient, she was worried that would negatively impact her healthcare (@Permanentlypis1 (1)(2)(3)).

This is a concern I've heard many times, from women who have both discussed their predicament publicly, as well as the women who wrote to me in confidence, after trying to engage their local hospitals in conversations about same-sex facilities and intimate care. In all cases, healthcare establishments either accused them of "bigotry" or minimised their concerns, and they routinely failed to guarantee access to same-sex clinicians and facilities. As a consequence, women either self-excluded from receiving healthcare, sometimes despite chronic health conditions, or they were intimidated into silence due to fears that the hospital would refuse to treat them.

Although such concerns may seem far-fetched, women who requested female-only care have indeed been denied treatment by hospitals. In one particularly shocking case, a female patient who was due to have a specialised procedure at Princess Grace Hospital in London, requested access to single-sex toilet facilities and that she not be asked to fill out paperwork about her "gender identity" as she did not believe in gender ideology. During a pre-operative assessment, which included an intimate procedure, a trans-identified male nurse entered the room uninvited, which this patient found intimidating and disconcerting. This prompted her to report a Patient Privacy Breach to the hospital, and to request that during her post-operative recovery, which would involve a week of being immobile, her intimate care be delivered by female nurses. In response, the hospital cancelled her procedure without any discussion with her, stating that they "did not share her beliefs", that they could not adhere to her requests and that they were "committed to protecting their staff from unacceptable distress" (Sales, 2022).

Medical students are being conditioned to accept this, using a mixture of ideological indoctrination and threat to their future careers. They are compelled to undergo training about "hate crimes", where they are told they can be expelled for "inappropriate behaviour" which, according to some of the modules, includes a "belief/insistence that transwomen are not real women".

Over the years that I've been writing about these issues, I've been contacted by many students and clinicians from all over the English-speaking world, all of whom were keen to discuss this, but only in confidence. Other conversations were held in public, on social media.

I would like to present a small selection of examples that illustrate the degree of concern and upset at the ideological coercion these clinicians are experiencing at their places of work and study. I have referenced the comments that were made in public. Others, which were shared with me privately with permission to include them on my website and in this book, are reproduced verbatim:

. . .

"Oh it's quite crazy over here! I'd rather not divulge the precise location but I can say it is an upper tier school with heavy involvement in research and teaching. Most of the wildest wokeness tends to be centered around race and gender – specifically, transgender ideology."

"In a journal club, when our group was drafting a problem statement for our patient (a girl with sickle cell disease), we wasted over 5 minutes debating whether it was appropriate to allude to the patient's sex in our opening statement. I argued that it was potentially relevant (I's not a sickle cell expert, but I suspect that sex might have some influence on disease severity), but the vocal minority in my group argued that 'we can only infer the patient's gender identity through her pronouns, we can't infer her assigned sex at birth, so we should just leave it out'. And keep in mind, all these examples are from "bread and butter" science classes. NOT the woo-woo gender identity materials and race relations workshops through which we also had to suffer."

"If any socially liberal/woke people ever try to say, 'Well, no one actually is saying that sex isn't real, they're just saying that gender is fluid', they are lying or misinformed. I was told this information on many, many separate occasions."

One student shared with me a video of a talk by a medical student, which was a part of official Hull York Medical School Pride month events and platformed on the medical school's social media pages. In this talk, a student tells her story in the third person, about a girl named Jessica who didn't feel comfortable with dresses, toys and other traditionally feminine activities. She describes being bullied, and later on in high school, realising that she was a lesbian. Soon afterwards, she was introduced to gender ideology online, including to the concept of being transgender. She went to university, changed her fashion style and even tried to be "hyper feminine" but apparently no matter what she did, it didn't feel right to her. Eventually she developed mental health problems and one night, under the stars, she told her friends, "I am not Jessica. I never felt like Jessica. I'm not a girl. I'm a man. William was born". This student's goal is to one day become a transgender medicine consultant (@hullyorkmed, 2020).

"In an anatomy lab where we were looking at a (disassembled?) pelvis/reproductive organs, I was asked 'Would you like to see the assigned-female-at-birth or the assigned-male-at-birth specimen first?'"

"Different prevalence of asthma between the sexes are 'most likely due to the difference in average ribcage size and not due to the gender of the people' (a very bold claim)."

"It was implied in a lecture that the different rates of cardiovascular disease in men vs women are actually due solely to the higher presence of androgens 'associated with AMAB people' and not 'easily dividable by sex'. Oh, by the way, biological sex is a social construct. That made my jaw drop to the floor."

. . .

"Many/most of the lecture and reader materials have been changed to say "AFAB" and "AMAB" or "XX individuals" and "XY individuals", in lieu of female and male. Most of the instructors don't seem to be super on-board with these distinctions but many are well-intentioned, trying to be polite/an "ally". If anything, this makes them much more vulnerable to scrutiny. I'm not sure if it's due to sexism or due to displays of weakness/appeasement, but the female professors who have committed Wrongspeak have been held to much higher scrutiny by my fellow uber-woke students than the male professors. We had a genetics professor who interchanged between using the terms "AFAB/AMAB" and "female/male" multiple times. In response, some of the wokest students drafted a 5-7 page letter outlining every one of her "crimes" and sent it around our class's Slack channel to get it signed and sent to the Deans so she could be encouraged to "do better" (ugh). I can recall three or four other petitions circulated for similar reasons, all related to similar instances."

Particularly concerning is biological sex denialism in midwifery and obstetrics and gynaecology education. One student recounted a bizarre discrepancy between the OB/GYN didactic course for her masters degree and her work experience. Although one fifth of her course material focused on trans-identifying males (transwomen) and there was no mention of postmenopausal women at all, half the patients she encountered during her clinical rotation were post-menopausal women while none were trans-identifying males. As her course focused on "inclusivity", the students were told that "not every woman has a vagina" and that they "should not refuse to do a Pap smear on a trans woman". This was justified by saying that, depending on the type of "bottom surgery" trans-identifying males have had, the clinician should check for appropriate tissue cancer (for example penile cancer in cases of penile inversion). However, hormone replacement for post-menopausal women was not covered at all, which attracted a complaint from one student (@RebeccPlum, 2021 (1) (2) (3)).

This is not an isolated incident. Napier University in Edinburgh updated its course guide on catheterisation by replacing the word "women" with "birthing people" and claiming that because biological males can get pregnant, student midwives should learn how to catheterise a penis.

They explained it by saying: "This update was made to take account of the fact that while most times the birthing person will have female genitalia, you may be caring for a pregnant or birthing person who is transitioning from male to female and may still have external male genitalia. You need to be familiar with the catheterisation procedure for both the female and male anatomy. For this reason, where appropriate, this book refers to the person or birthing person" (Wade, 2022).

To be clear, men cannot get pregnant regardless of how they identify, because their sex is male and instead of ovaries and a uterus - which are female reproductive organs - they have penises and testicles. There's never been a successful case of uterine implantation into a man, let alone a case of such an implanted uterus successfully carrying a pregnancy. Therefore, teaching midwives to catheterise a male penis is redundant.

If we give the guidance authors the benefit of the doubt, it is possible that they confused "trans women" (men who identify as women), with "trans men" (women who identify as men).

Trans-identifying females ("trans men") can undertake a

variety of gender-reassignment interventions, some of which are compatible with pregnancy - such as social transition and cross-sex hormones - and some are not - such as removal of the vagina and creation of a neo-phallus.

A neo-phallus is a surgically created, non-functional appendage fashioned from a flap of tissue wrapped around an artificial "erectile prosthesis" which can be manually inflated to allow for penetrative intercourse. In the course of these procedures, the female urethra can be diverted to the perineum or artificially lengthened in order to create a functional penile urethra. All these procedures have a high complication rate, and urethral lengthening in particular can result in strictures and fistulas. Therefore, catheterising trans-identifying females who have had phalloplasty usually requires specialist input and equipment, and when this isn't readily available, clinicians tend to opt for suprapubic catheterisation (directly into the bladder just above the pubic area).

Another thing worth mentioning is that phalloplasty in females is preceded by a hysterectomy (and often oophorectomy), which makes it extremely unlikely that a trans-identifying female with a neo-phallus would ever need midwifery care, and even if she did, midwives would be ill-equipped to catheterise such a patient if they relied on their knowledge of male anatomy.

These examples illustrate the pitfalls of so called "gender neutral" language, which typically amounts to the erasure of female-specific terminology. Whenever you see material claiming that a female-specific illness or physiological process happens to "birthing people", "menstruators" or "vulva owners", you will find equivalent material that talks about male-specific physiology and disease affecting "men" and "boys", not "ejaculators", "impregnators" and "penis owners".

While medical institutions insist that this misogyny is motivated by a desire to include women who identify as men, in reality, healthcare staff and students are coerced into going along with it. As one student midwife shared, unless she uses the phrase "birthing people" to describe pregnant women in her papers, she gets "docked" (@Chelsie63556770, 2021).

In a sea of bad examples, some institutions are trying to ethically navigate the gender reassignment minefield, such as one medical school which staged an OSCE station with a trans-identifying patient and marked the students on both using the patient's preferred pronouns as well as noting the patient's biological sex. This is an essential skill future clinicians need to learn, in order to establish rapport with their trans-identifying patients and to diagnose and treat them appropriately.

The overwhelming picture, however, is one of both students and clinicians operating in an environment saturated with gender ideology.

Clinical practice

Despite, arguably, the best intentions of those who are promoting gender ideology in medicine, these policies also compromise the medical care of the very people they are supposed to protect, as this example given to me by a clinician working in the Emergency Department illustrates:

"I saw a transwoman in the ED the other day. Medical records all said 'female'. NHS number was new. Nothing from the patient to reveal natal sex, except 'I take HRT'. I could see this patient was taking 6x the exogenous oral oestrogen normally taken post-menopause, plus a weekly patch. Formerly took androgen blocker used in feminisation therapy for males, and had had NHS speech and language therapy.

With patient's consent I viewed the Summary Care Records

(SCR) to record drug history accurately in the notes. In the SCR natal sex was not recorded. All it contained was childhood immunisations and current drugs. No 'diagnosis' relating to drug history. No record of any surgery.

A few points.

If this patient was bleeding, I would send group and save [blood sample processing that determines the patient's blood group and screens for any atypical antibodies]. This would go to blood bank with sex erroneously marked as female. I'm not a haematologist but are there risks around this I don't know?

If the patient donated blood, is natal sex recorded?

Patient had shortness of breath/cough/chest pain. Was sent in for PE [pulmonary embolism - blood clot in lung] work-up, presumably because the massive doses of oestrogen are a big risk factor.

I did bloods, d-dimer, chest X ray etc.

Investigations were negative for PE but there was an incidental finding on chest x-ray of healed fractures with no history of trauma, which is unusual to see in a young patient.

I was concerned this might indicate reduced bone density, knowing this can be a side-effect of gender reassignment therapy. I discussed this with the patient, without at any point suggesting that I didn't take patient's recorded sex at face value. I thought it was in the patient's best interest to mention the incidental finding in the patient's discharge letter.

Anyway, I'm telling you all this because I suppose it highlighted to me a few things about how unhelpful it is from a clinical point of view to go down this gender rabbit hole. For the patient, passing and being dissociated from their natal sex is important. They are permitted to have a new name, NHS number and sex on their records. Their wish/need for gender affirmation is prioritised over their clinician knowing something as fundamental as their sex when it comes to diagnosing and treating them.

Also, the current climate means that, presented with a patient like this, I can tell you I was nervous as hell about saying the wrong thing. I'm not talking about misgendering, it's easy not to do that. What I mean was that I was terrified of saying anything that hinted I'd observed or considered that the patient might be a transwoman, in case I upset them or attracted a complaint.

There was lack of candour and openness, and wariness on both sides, which is not conducive to delivering best clinical care to the patient.

Prior to this encounter I was unaware you could change both your sex and NHS number on your records. I looked into it and I found a discussion on Reddit between some young trans individuals who were exchanging information about how to get a new NHS number (from what I remember it is easy and I'm not even convinced you need a GRC).

What was also clear, is that their priority in getting new NHS number is so they can actually hide, erase, their sex... it's all about passing."

We already know that serious medical errors caused by mis-sexing are affecting trans-identified patients. One of the essays in this book analyses a case of a trans-identified female being denied renal transplant because the medical team kept using male equations to calculate her renal function.

There is another well-publicised case of a trans-identified female presenting to the Emergency Department with abdominal pain. Although this patient told the medical team she was transgender, that she had had a positive result with an at home pregnancy test and that she "peed herself" - which could be a sign of imminent labour - her medical notes had a male sex marker. Instead of recognising that the patient was in the late stages of pregnancy, the nurse decided the patient was "obese" and didn't triage her appropriately. The patient ended up delivering a stillborn baby (Marchione, 2019).

Both these cases occurred despite the medical team knowing the true sex of the patient. Now imagine an all-too likely scenario of a well-passing trans-identifying patient who doesn't inform the medical team of their sex. The risk of medical errors is simply unacceptable.

Data about patients' biological sex has been seriously compromised by health services replacing "sex" with "gender" and "gender identity", and by entertaining a preposterous notion that biological sex is arbitrarily "assigned at birth" and therefore changeable. As a result of pretending that biological sex is either a feeling or the imitation of masculine or feminine gender stereotypes, single-sex categories have been replaced with mixed sex categories, where women, girls and trans-identifying males are now categorised as having "female gender" while men, boys and trans-identifying females are categorised as having "male gender".

This is how the twenty-week ultrasound scans pregnant women in the UK receive as a part of their antenatal screening have been rebranded as "gender scans" (@Ashworth, 2020), while breast cancer related questionnaires in the United States ask patients what sex they were "assigned at birth" in order to be more "inclusive" (@Beatthemedian, 2020).

It took months of campaigning by women to get Irish cervical screening material to include the word "woman" alongside "people with a cervix", but it still completely omits the word "female". This has led to muddled, borderline misleading statements such as "Every year in Ireland about 300 people get cervical cancer. 90 women die from it."

This is despite surveys showing most women don't know what a cervix is (Bakar, 2020) and that many are unaware of the screening at all (BBC, 2017).

Following further complaints from women and health professionals, this has now been amended to "Every year in Ireland about 290 women get cervical cancer. Almost 90 of those women die from it" (HSE, 2021).

One would have thought that the Covid-19 pandemic, and the fact that males are at greater risk of severe outcomes, would have motivated health services to stop this charade and start collecting data on biological sex. Unfortunately, this is not the case. People who are asked to fill out Covid-19 related questionnaires (either for the purpose of assessing health and safety at work or before participating in a Covid-19 antibody trials) report being asked "What gender are you? Male, female, non-binary or other" (@fergusrabbit, 2020), and having to explain to healthcare professionals that Covid-19 affects sexes differently and that the virus doesn't care about a person's gender identity (@DarlinBudsOfMeh).

Perhaps most shocking of all is the fact that NHS Blood and Transplant also don't collect accurate information on biological sex from prospective donors. Instead, those signing up to donate blood are asked whether their "gender" is male or female, and those signing up for organ donation are asked, "On my GP records, I am recorded as: Male, Female or Neither matches my GP record".

When Clare B. Dimyon MBE (@BDimyon) asked NHS Organ Donation why they used gender instead of sex on sign up forms, they stated that potential donors could "choose from the following options when it comes to selecting a gender online: Male, Female, Transgender, Other, Prefer Not To Say." (@NHSOrganDonor, 2021 (1)))

Blood donors on Twitter reacted by pointing out that this service used to ask for biological sex in the past. They wondered how the NHS Organ Donation service records donor sex now and why they aren't asking for medically relevant information that is based on material reality (@Freakiest14, 2021).

"Male and female are sexes. Being transgender isn't a sex, or even a 'gender'. It could mean a variety of things." (@Rhyw-Fenyw, 2021)

When pressed repeatedly about the potential for medical errors if gender, rather than sex, is recorded, @NHSOrganDonor claimed that when opting in for organ donation, biological sex "is not an essential piece of information". However, at the point of organ matching, sex would apparently be considered alongside other medical, travel and social history, and this information would be retrieved from the patient's medical notes. (@NHSOrganDonor, 2021 (2), (3); NHS Blood and Transplant, 2021)

Unfortunately, as demonstrated previously, when trans-identifying patients request a change of sex marker on their medical records, a new NHS number is issued and all the information relating to their biological sex (erroneously referred to as "previous gender identity") is removed.

Considering that men have been reported to experience severe adverse reactions from receiving blood and plasma from women, and that a sex mismatch between donor and recipient could contribute to increased rejection and complication rates of organ transplant procedures, mis-sexing in this context is not only unwise, it is potentially clinically negligent (Zimmerman & McGregor, 2020).

Medical insurance

In a document titled *Permissibility of denial of coverage based solely on age for female-to-male chest reconstruction surgery as part of a treatment for gender dysphoria,* the California Department of Insurance offered a legal opinion that an insurer may not deny coverage for mastectomy for female patients undergoing gender reassignment, solely based on the patient's age (Schnoll, 2020).

They cited WPATH standards of care, which claimed that mastectomies and "creation of a male chest" were a "medically necessary surgical treatment of gender dysphoria for female-to-male patients who meet specific criteria". According to this document, "the presence of female chest" in females who identify as males "is an abnormal body structure caused by gender dysphoria" and mastectomies are performed to "correct or repair abnormal structures of the body caused by congenital defects, developmental abnormalities, trauma, infection, tumors, or disease". This is apparently designed to "create a normal appearance, to the extent possible in an individual transitioning from female to male".

This is how, by pathologising normal female anatomy in girls who identify as the opposite sex, cosmetic mastectomies are reframed as "medically necessary" and therefore covered by insurance.

At the time this document was written, WPATH recommended "age of majority" as a criterion for surgical gender reassignment procedures, but emphasised that mastectomies could be carried out earlier, "depending on an adolescent's specific clinical situation and goals for gender identity expression."

When WPATH guidelines were updated in September 2022, minimum ages for medical and surgical gender reassignment procedures were removed from the original document without explanation (Coleman, et al., 2022; Statement of Removal, 2022).

In Australia, on the other hand, the prescribing of testosterone is listed in the Pharmaceutical Benefits Scheme. This means that the Australian government subsidises the cost of this medicine. However the indications do not include "transgender hormonal management", which means that masculinising hormone therapy for women who identify as men is not covered. This is because testosterone manufacturers haven't done studies specifically on trans-identifying female patients, nor did they apply to the Pharmaceutical Benefits Advisory Committee to get testosterone approved for use in this patient population.

Some Australian doctors are circumventing this by claiming that "transgender men are males" who have low testosterone and androgen deficiency due to missing testicles, and they are using the indication of "androgen deficiency due to an established testicular disorder" to prescribe masculinising doses of testosterone to women who identify as men (Swannell, 2019),

Experimental surgery on transgender individuals

In a research study proposal titled 'Male to Female Transgender women's perceptions to womb transplantation', Womb Transplant UK informed prospective participants that this study "seeks to gain greater understanding of the desire, and therefore need, to perform womb transplantation as part of gender reassignment surgery." It went on to discuss recent successes in transplanting wombs into female patients, before veering off into speculation about how this could be done in males (Smith, 2018).

This particular demographic - men who identify as women - were "invited to participate because you are a male to female (M2F) transgender woman. You therefore have absolute uterine factor infertility (AUFI), a condition that affects one in 500 women of childbearing age."

This makes about as much sense as diagnosing humans with "absolute wing factor flightlessness" for the purposes of a study to explore human attitudes to wing transplants from albatrosses. Furthermore, because a uterus is not a part of male anatomy, attempting to surgically insert a uterus into a male body should be referred to as uterine implantation, not "transplantation".

This study has now been published under the title 'Perceptions and Motivations for Uterus Transplant in Transgender Women', with the following conclusion:

"In this study, transgender women reported a desire to have physiologic experiences unique to cisgender women, such as menstruation and gestation, as well as potentially having a physiologically functioning transplanted vagina. Our findings suggest that some transgender women may believe the potential benefits of uterus transplant outweigh the significant risks with which it is associated and may improve quality of life, happiness, and dysphoric symptoms while enhancing feelings of femininity. As such, just as the desire to experience gestation and psychological sequelae spurred uterus transplant research in women categorized as female at birth with AUFI, uterus transplant in transgender women could be considered in the same light, and research should be undertaken regarding its feasibility" (Jones, et al., 2021).

It is not ethical for clinicians to ignore sex differences between males and females, regardless of the context. However, in this proposed scenario - implanting a uterus into a man for the purpose of him carrying a pregnancy - the stakes are even higher.

It is not just adult men who arguably cannot consent to being harmed by unnecessary experimentation such as this. In an unlikely scenario that the implanted uterus is capable of gestating a pregnancy, the consequences to the human foetus, who would be exposed to a cocktail of drugs - including immunosuppressants - are unacceptable. There is no discussion about this, however. The references to the male "desire" to be pregnant are taken on face value and the language which seeks to obscure their male sex is used to reach the conclusion that just because in rare instances, uterine transplantation helped a woman carry a pregnancy, men who identify as women should be afforded the same experience.

Men who identify as women often have desires to experience physiological functions that are unique to female bodies. These desires are sometimes motivated by the irrational belief that they were "born in the wrong body", and other times, they are motivated by autogynaephilia - a paraphilic disorder whereby a biological male is aroused at a thought of himself as a female. This paraphilia ranges anywhere from a desire to cross-dress and impersonate a woman socially, to a desire to experience pregnancy, abortion, breastfeeding and menstruation. In the past, autogynaephilia was categorised as a gender identity disorder and transvestic fetish, and it has only been recategorised as "gender dysphoria" and a "human right to self-expression" under the intense pressure from transactivists. Despite this, there is no compelling scientific evidence that adult males who identify as women and who have an intense desire to experience pregnancy, are no longer psychologically vulnerable or afflicted with a paraphilic disorder.

The co-ordinator of this study published another article titled 'Uterine Transplantation in Transgender Women' in 2018 (Jones, et al, 2018).

In it, he mentions ethics but only in so far as asserting that performing uterine "transplants" in men who identify as women is motivated by "considerations of justice and equality". He goes on to equate men who identify as women with actual women, and likens men's distress at not being fertile as females, with women's distress at being infertile.

This paper invokes the Equality Act 2010 in order to claim that not offering uterine implantation to men who identify as women is direct and indirect discrimination against the protected characteristic of "gender reassignment". This is yet another example of an erroneous interpretation of the Equality Act, which underpins a lot of the cognitive and ideological capture of the medical profession by gender identity ideology.

Diagnosis of "absolute uterine factor infertility" in trans-identifying patients, and the just and equal access to treatment for this condition, can only reasonably apply to females who identify as males (otherwise known as "transgender men" or "female-to-male transsexuals"), who were either born with anatomical abnormalities causing infertility or who've had their uteruses removed as a part of surgical gender reassignment.

Refusing to consider these females for uterine transplants purely because they identify as male, would indeed constitute discrimination based on the protected characteristic of "gender reassignment". But this is not what is being proposed at all. Instead, trans-identifying female patients are seen as a source of female reproductive organs and pawns in dubious ethical arguments that propose surgical experiments on trans-identifying males (Api, et al., 2017).

Conclusion

There are many examples of institutional and cognitive capture of the medical profession by the pseudoscientific ideology which posits that some people were "born in the wrong body" and that the role of the clinician is to affirm and facilitate this belief.

Our ability to provide best medical care to patients - especially women and people who identify as transgender - as well as the integrity and ethics of the medical profession itself, has therefore been undermined, and it will take a joint effort from many clinicians, politicians and members of the public to put a stop to this.

Having said that, it is unacceptable that the burden of addressing the issue of biology denialism in the medical profession has fallen on patients. The longer the medical establishment and individual clinicians remain silent, the more severely compromised doctor-patient relationships and public trust in the medical profession will become. Therefore, I hope this book serves as a call to action.

Bibliography

Nolan, I.T. Kuhner, C.J. & Dy, G.W. (2019). Demographic and temporal trends in transgender identities and gender confirming surgery. Translational andrology and urology, 8(3), 184–190. https://doi.org/10.21037/tau.2019.04.09

Stonewall UK. (2015). Women and Equalities Select Committee Inquiry on Transgender Equality. https://www.stonewall.org.uk/cy/node/9461

Stonewall UK. (2020) Stonewall statement on Tavistock appeal. https://www.stonewall.org.uk/about-us/news/stonewall-statement-tavistock-appeal

Sex Matters. (2021). Stonewall Champions List - We have written to all 850 Stonewall Champions and are tracking who has left. https://sex-matters.org/stonewall-champions-list/

GMC. (no date (1)). Maintain your registration. https://www.gmc-uk.org/registration-and-licensing/managing-your-registration/information-for-doctors-on-the-register/maintain-your-registration

PCSE. (no date). Process for registering a patient gender re-assignment. pcse.england.nhs.uk. https://pcse.england.nhs.uk/media/1291/process-for-registering-a-patient-gender-re-assignment.pdf

LGBT Foundation. (2020). Changing a patient's name and gender marker. https://www.weobleyandstauntonsurgeries.nhs.uk/website/M81018/files/Changing%20Your%20name%20and%20Gender%20with%20the%20NHS.pdf

GMC. (no date (2)). Trans healthcare. https://www.gmc-uk.org/ethical-guidance/ethical-hub/trans-healthcare#Confidentiality%20and%20equality

GMC. (no date (3)). How to make your practice more inclusive. https://www.gmc-uk.org/ethical-guidance/ethical-hub/trans-healthcare#Trans%20healthcare

Lancaster Guardian. (2018). Lancaster mum with 'fear of men' locked on hospital ward with transgender patient. https://www.lancasterguardian.co.uk/news/lancaster-mum-fear-men-locked-hospital-ward-transgender-patient-653048

Beal, J. (2022). Hospital 'dismissed claim of rape by trans attacker'. The Times. https://www.thetimes.co.uk/article/hospital-dismissed-claim-of-rape-by-trans-attacker-bssxvbqch

Trueland, J. (2020). Push for progress on transgender rights in healthcare. The BMA. https://www.bma.org.uk/news-and-opinion/push-for-progress-on-transgender-rights-in-healthcare

Carmichael, P. Butler, G. Masic, U. Cole, T. J. De Stavola, B. L. Davidson, S. Skageberg, E. M. Khadr, S. Viner, R. M. (2021). Short-term outcomes of pubertal suppression in a selected cohort of 12 to 15 year old young people with persistent gender dysphoria in the UK. Plos One. https://doi.org/10.1371/journal.pone.0243894

Bowen, M. Clyde, K. Wright, E. Katz, T. Hakeem, A. Griffin, L. Re: Gender dysphoria service rated inadequate after waiting list of 4600 raises concerns. The BMJ. https://www.bmj.com/content/372/bmj.n205/rr-0

Chisholm, J. (2021). BMA response to Dr Bowen, Dr Clyde, Dr Wright et al. https://www.bmj.com/content/372/bmj.n205/rr-3

BMA. (2020). BMA submission: Women and Equalities Committee inquiry on Reform of the Gender Recognition Act. https://www.bma.org.uk/media/3584/bma-submission-reform-of-the-gender-recognition-act.pdf

@CareQualityComm. (2020). There's nothing in Act that says that we need to use a specific word for a protected characteristic. When we use gender as a descriptor of one of the protected characteristics (as we do in equality monitoring form), there's no evidence to show that we are excluding anyone (2/3). Twitter. 17 Sep, 2020. https://twitter.com/CareQualityComm/status/1306560421982330880

Forstater, M. (2020). Trans healthcare professionals and patient consent. https://a-question-of-consent.net/2020/09/16/doctors/

CQC. (2016). East One Health Quality Report. https://api.cqc.org.uk/public/v1/reports/377f483b-4528-4da7-bbc6-c6ba20782359

CQC. (2017). East One Health Quality Report. https://api.cqc.org.uk/public/v1/reports/78f9b366-a5c6-4df3-ac8f-f93b59cee46a

CQC. (2018). Sexual safety on mental health wards. https://www.cqc.org.uk/publications/major-report/sexual-safety-mental-health-wards

Medical Schools Council, (2021). Athena SWAN. https://www.medschools.ac.uk/our-work/equality-diversity-inclusion/athena-swan

Advance HE. (2020). Gender Equality Guidance. https://www.advance-he.ac.uk/sites/default/files/2020-04/20%20Gender%20Equality%20Guidance%20v1%20Mar%2020.pdf

Pugh, E. (2016). Trans staff and students in HE and colleges: improving experiences. Formerly available at: https://s3.eu-west-2.amazonaws.com/assets.creode.advancehe-document-manager/documents/ecu/TransguidanceMay20171579704782.pdf - now removed. Updated version (2022)

available at: https://s3.eu-west-2.amazonaws.com/assets.creode.advancehe-document-manager/documents/advance-he/Trans_staff%20and%20students_HE_guidance_1655287866.pdf or https://drive.google.com/file/d/1SBximrNW-Var09p6Nu0RyXCLu9fnOE_0/view?usp=sharing

Equality Challenge Unit. (2016). Trans equality policy statement. Formerly available at: https://s3.eu-west-2.amazonaws.com/assets.creode.advancehe-document-manager/documents/ecu/Trans-equality-policy-statement1579088209.pdf - now removed. Screenshots of relevant pages available at: https://drive.google.com/file/d/1T5MSdwJMwinFSJwz-Q-X9GwzN4cOBXFH/view?usp=sharing

@Permanentlypis1. (2021 (1)). Had my 1st experience in the 1st lockdown, finally built enough courage to tell my gp why a colonoscopy was such a difficult procedure to subject myself to but was reassured, had a general, came round to a trans identified male nurse pinning me down I was completely freaked out! Twitter. 5 Jan, 2021. https://twitter.com/Permanentlypis1/status/1346534677302145027

@Permanentlypis1. (2021(2)). Yes I did because I have urge incontinence and knew if I was out for the count I was going to wet myself and would need changing. Twitter. 5 Jan, 2020. https://twitter.com/Permanentlypis1/status/1346537379339923457

@Permanentlypis1. (2021 (3)). Thanks, Tbh I thought of nothing else afterwards but I don't trust the Trust or the NHS not to treat me as the problem and as someone with chronic conditions I don't need anything else to negatively impact my care. Twitter. 5 Jan, 2020. https://twitter.com/Permanentlypis1/status/1346553478466981895

Sales, D. (2022). EXCLUSIVE: Hospital refuses to operate on sex attack victim after she requests all-female care because she fears mixed sex facilities are unsafe for women. Daily Mail. https://www.dailymail.co.uk/news/article-11316141/Hospital-bans-sex-assault-victim-op-female-care-request.html

@hullyorkmed (2020). Pride 2020. Instagram. https://www.instagram.com/tv/CBh7sOUnNLW/?utm_medium=copy_link

@RebeccPlum. (2021 (1)). During my OB/GYN didactic course for my masters degree. 1/5th of the course concentrated on trans women, that's 20% of the course work focused on biological males, 0% on post menopausal women. Yet, my rotation (real life) 0 trans patients and 55% post menopausal women. Twitter. Mar 20, 2021. https://twitter.com/RebeccPlum/status/1373081035949404166

@RebeccPlum. (2021 (2)). Yes, please do. I should clarify that we also covered STDs during this course. (I just want to be as honest as possible).

The first week of a 7 wk course was on inclusivity, how not every woman has a vagina....We were told we should not refuse to do a Pap on a trans woman...." Twitter. Mar 20, 2021. https://twitter.com/RebeccPlum/status/1373385099308318725

@RebeccPlum. (2021 (3)) In trans women who have had bottom surgery depending on the type of surgery we should check for that type tissue cancer (ie penile cancer). And we DID NOT cover post menopausal hormone replacement in fact one student even complained about that in my clinical rotation group. Twitter. Mar 20, 2021. https://twitter.com/RebeccPlum/status/1373386245376765956

Wade, M. (2022). Student midwives at Napier University taught that men can get pregnant - Online module had guide to catheterising 'birthing people' with penises. The Sunday Times. https://www.thetimes.co.uk/article/student-midwives-at-napier-university-taught-that-men-can-get-pregnant-bsxvjodcp

@Chelsie63556770. (2021). I am a midwifery student. I have to use "pregnant people" in my papers or I get docked. Twitter. Jan 4, 2021. https://twitter.com/Chelsie63556770/status/1345976055039856641

Marchione, M. (2019). Nurse mistakes pregnant transgender man as obese. Then, the man births a stillborn baby. USA Today. https://eu.usatoday.com/story/news/health/2019/05/16/pregnant-transgender-man-births-stillborn-baby-hospital-missed-labor-signs/3692201002/

@Ashworth101. (2020). Someone I know had her 20 week baby scan yesterday (UK) It's now called a gender scan... Not sure when that changed. Twitter. Dec 28, 2020. https://twitter.com/Ashworth101/status/1343572241775271937

@Beatthemedian. (2020). This is worrying. I was filling out a breast cancer related questionnaire (American) and it asked me what sex I was assigned at birth. The very nice woman who designed it was trying to be kind and inclusive. Let's stick to reality and facts when it comes to healthcare FFS. [quoted tweet] Twitter. Dec 28, 2020. https://twitter.com/Beatthemedian/status/1343602950506237956

Bakar, F. (2020). Almost 50% of women don't know where their cervix or uterus is, nor the purpose of menstruation, study finds. https://metro.co.uk/2020/11/09/almost-50-of-women-dont-know-where-their-cervix-is-finds-study-13561743/

BBC. (2017). No-show women at cervical screening 'unaware of test'. https://www.bbc.co.uk/news/health-40444170

HSE. (2021). Cervical cancer - Overview. https://www2.hse.ie/conditions/cervical-cancer/overview/

@fergusrabbit. (2020). Taking part in a Covid antibody research trial. They are not recording sex. They asked - What gender are you? - male, female, Non-binary, other. Really don't see the point in them asking at all. When they start doing this in medical research, you know the world has gone to shit.Twitter. Dec 20, 2020. https://twitter.com/fergusrabbit/status/1343667177728200704

@DarlinBudsOfMeh. (2021). This stuff is so annoying. I completed a Covid survey recently for the HSE and they asked for my gender (with myriad options). I explained to them that covid affects the sexes differently; it doesn't care about the person's gender identity. Twitter. Jan 6, 2021. https://twitter.com/DarlinBudsOfMeh/status/1346784126377074688

@NHSOrganDonor. (2021 (1)). Hi Clare. You can choose from the following options when it comes to selecting a gender online: Male, Female, Transgender, Other, Prefer Not To Say. You can also register a decision on the Organ Donor Register via our 24hr helpline on 0300 123 23 23. Twitter. Jan 5, 2021. https://twitter.com/NHSOrganDonor/status/1346483687819517954

@Freakiest14. (2021). When I opted in years ago, I was told to select my sex. Why is it now different? Nothing has changed between then and now. Women are still female and men are still male. Everything else is personality and makes no difference to their organs. Twitter. Jan 6, 2021 (deleted tweet)

@RhywFenyw. (2021). How do you register your sex? Everyone has a biological sex. Why aren't you asking for information that is actually medically relevant and based on material reality? Male and female are sexes. Being transgender isn't a sex, or even a 'gender'. It could mean a variety of things. Twitter. Jan 9, 2021. https://twitter.com/RhywFenyw/status/1347851712674017280

@NHSOrganDonor. (2021 (2)). In registering a decision to opt-in, this is not an essential piece of information, however when it comes to organ matching, sex, along with medical, travel and social history are considered. We hope this helps - Patrick. Twitter. Jan 6, 2021. https://twitter.com/NHSOrganDonor/status/1346787852567408640

@NHSOrganDonor. (2021 (3)). This info would come from your medical history/notes which is checked before any donation takes place. Family support also helps make sure that vital info is available to understand whether a person's organs are safe to transplant into somebody else - Patrick.

Twitter. Jan 6, 2021. https://twitter.com/NHSOrganDonor/status/1346825033478508544

NHS Blood and Transplant. (2021). Statement on how gender is currently requested on the NHS Organ Donor Register. https://www.organdonation.nhs.uk/get-involved/news/statement-on-how-gender-is-currently-requested-on-the-nhs-organ-donor-register/

Zimmerman, B. J. McGregor, A. J. (2020). Sex- and Gender-Related Factors in Blood Product Transfusions. Gender and the Genome. Volume 4: 1-5. DOI:10.1177/2470289720948064 https://www.researchgate.net/publication/344975951_Sex-_and_Gender-Related_Factors_in_Blood_Product_Transfusions

Schnoll, K. B. (2020). Permissibility of denial of coverage based solely on age for female-to-male chest reconstruction surgery as part of a treatment for gender dysphoria. https://www.insurance.ca.gov/0250-insurers/0300-insurers/0200-bulletins/bulletin-notices-commiss-opinion/upload/Gender-dysphoria-male-chest-surgery-CDI-GC-opinion-letter-12-30-20.pdf

Coleman, E. Radix, A. E. Bouman, W. P. et al. (2022). Standards of Care for the Health of Transgender and Gender Diverse People, Version 8, International Journal of Transgender Health, 23:sup1, S1-S259, DOI:10.1080/26895269.2022.2100644 https://www.tandfonline.com/doi/pdf/10.1080/26895269.2022.2100644

(2022) Statement of Removal, International Journal of Transgender Health, 23:sup1, S259, DOI: 10.1080/26895269.2022.2125695 https://www.tandfonline.com/doi/full/10.1080/26895269.2022.2125695

Swannell, C. (2019). Empowering GPs to care for transgender patients. https://insightplus.mja.com.au/2019/30/empowering-gps-to-care-for-transgender-patients/?fbclid=IwAR0lWCBmDeAVGEUOulCnNu39PvN31f4womjee3ZUwrcz15vAyzbOco7s8HA

Smith, R. (2018). Male to Female Transgender women's perceptions to womb transplantation - Participant Information Sheet (V3 - 21/11/2018). https://drive.google.com/file/d/1iq-chQ_9munOClW4S3MMi9HcdllsdY24/view?usp=sharing

Jones, B.P. Rajamanoharan, A. Vali, S. et al. (2021). Perceptions and Motivations for Uterus Transplant in Transgender Women. JAMA Netw Open. 4(1):e2034561. doi:10.1001/jamanetworkopen.2020.34561 https://jamanetwork.com/journals/jamanetworkopen/fullarticle/2775302

Jones, B.P. Williams, N.J. Saso, S. Thum, M.Y. Quiroga, I. Yazbek, J. Wilkinson, S. Ghaem-Maghami, S. Thomas, P. & Smith, J.R. (2018). Uterine transplantation in transgender women. BJOG : an international journal of obstetrics and gynaecology, 126(2), 152–156. https://doi.org/10.1111/1471-0528.15438

Api, M. Boza, A. & Ceyhan, M. (2017). Could the female-to-male transgender population be donor candidates for uterus transplantation?. Turkish journal of obstetrics and gynecology, 14(4), 233–237. https://doi.org/10.4274/tjod.55453

Chapter 22

My Interview With FiLiA - A Feminist Doctor on Gender Identity Policies, Institutional Capture and Medicine (FiLiA, 2021)

La Scapigliata is a feminist writer and medical doctor. She is outspoken on the harms of gender identity policies, sharing medical expertise to debunk various myths and writing passionately in defense of women's sex-based rights. FiLiA caught up with her to discuss her work investigating how ideas prioritising the concept of gender identity have become embedded in various UK medical institutions.

What was your initial assessment of how medicine understands or manages patients who identify as other than their biological sex?

Working in psychiatry, I encountered several transsexuals who became acutely suicidal following sex-reassignment surgery. They were homosexual males with a diagnosis of Gender Identity Disorder (GID), who had undergone a thorough assessment and counselling to ensure their suitability for these procedures and to help them manage their expectations.

When their psychological distress didn't go away, following surgery, they described feeling mutilated and wanting their old bodies back. This was unfortunately not possible because these operations were irreversible. I had a great deal of empathy for these patients, but I also understood the impulse of a doctor to do something, anything, as a last resort to help alleviate a patient's distress at being born male. I wasn't convinced that sex-reassignment was the best way to go about achieving this, but I trusted my colleagues, who were experts in this area, to have solid science behind what they were doing.

When I started examining this issue in detail, I first wanted to familiarise myself with the scientific rationale for sex-reassignment. To my surprise, I couldn't find any studies that showed long-term improvements. Instead, the biggest study on sex-reassigned individuals (Dhejne et al 2011) showed significant increase in mortality, morbidity and suicide over time. Despite this, a whole new population of patients, mainly girls but also some boys, were being diagnosed with "gender dysphoria" and instead of being offered counselling, they were fast-tracked to a medical pathway (Evans 2021) and to a "gender reassignment" that involved hormone blockers, cross-sex hormones and eventually, irreversible surgeries such as double mastectomies, hysterectomies and surgical castration.

I looked up Gender Dysphoria (GD) (Zucker, 2015) and found that it had replaced GID in the diagnostic manual for psychiatrists (called DSM-V). The criteria appeared very similar in spirit, but the persistent discomfort with one's biological sex and identification with the opposite sex, that I have seen in my patients, was now redefined as a mismatch between one's "experienced/expressed gender," and "assigned gender."

The criteria never defines "gender," but judging by the

description of boys and girls as "assigned genders" it is safe to assume they are referring to biological sex.

But if this was the case, why do they also talk about "desire to be of the other gender (or some alternative gender different from assigned gender)"?

What did you think about the phrase "assigned gender" in this context?

Biological sex is binary and observed at birth with 99.98% accuracy (Hilton 2018). The remaining 0.02% of babies have Disorders of Sex Development (formerly known as intersex) (Sax 2002) and while they might need genetic testing to determine their biological sex, they are still either male or female. There are no other, or in-between, sexes.

In the past, children with DSDs were operated on in order to make their bodies appear more sex-typical, and sometimes, the decision was made to raise them as the opposite sex. This procedure was known as "assigning sex," but because we know that the socialisation of males and females is heavily influenced by gender stereotypes, and that biological sex can't be changed, it could be argued that this constituted "assigning gender" instead. However, this language relates to a very specific, rare set of circumstances where doctors found it difficult to classify a child's sex based on "ambiguous" physical features, so medics may have "assigned" those children as girls or boys and surgically altered their genitalia to look more "normal." This practice is not the same as in 99.98% of cases, where doctors simply observe a child's biological sex and note it on a birth certificate.

The vast majority of children and adults who were diagnosed with GD were correctly, and easily, recognised as their biological sex at birth. We know this, because when doctors screened for DSDs in patients who have GD, they found it was very rare: the incidence of DSDs is the same as in the general population (Pang 2018).

Therefore it appeared that the terminology used to describe DSD patients' unique experiences was being misapplied to give an air of scientific legitimacy to a linguistically convoluted and scientifically imprecise diagnosis of gender dysphoria.

How does a feminist lens complement your understanding of the medical approach to gender dysphoria?

GD criteria talk a lot about gender stereotypes, which feminists consider to be socially constructed and designed to disadvantage females. Females are supposed to be submissive and perform free emotional, domestic and sexual labour (femininity) while males are supposed to be aggressive, dominant, and have a leading role in society (masculinity). Seen through this lens, it was easy to understand the surge in referrals of girls and young women to gender identity clinics, and how replacing "sex" with "gender" in the wording of the diagnosis shifted the narrative from distress with one's biological sex, to distress with gender non-conformance. But instead of advocating for greater acceptance of gender non-conformity, and offering counselling as the first-line treatment, with gender reassignment as a last resort, the treatment was changed to an "affirmative model", whereby patients' "gender identity" had to be validated by offering gender reassignment as the first-line treatment, while counselling was likened to "conversion therapy" and it fell out of favour.

This practice of "affirmation" has a particularly negative impact on women and girls, because most young patients with gender dysphoria in the UK now are females (Griffin 2020), who have other factors such as autism, sexual trauma or emerging homosexuality that could explain the discomfort they feel about their bodies and restrictive social norms.

The mantra of "affirmation without exception" is also used more broadly, to deny that females have different needs and experiences than males, to accuse women of being "exclusionary" for wanting to retain single-sex spaces and to portray males who identify as women/girls as "victims" of female boundaries.

What do you mean by gender identity policies, and to what degree do you think such ideas are scientifically sound?

Policies prioritising gender identity are based on a post-modern belief system that asserts the primacy of gender identity (one's internal sense of being male or female) over biological sex. When gender identity is congruent with biological sex the person is said to be "cisgender," and when it is incongruent, they are "transgender." This set of ideas around the concept of gender identity maintains an old-fashioned belief in traditional sex-roles, or gender stereotypes, but adds a modern twist to it. Women and girls are still "inherently feminine" and men and boys are "inherently masculine," but a man who likes to wear dresses and make up "could really be a woman," while a girl who hates dresses and likes to climb trees "could really be a boy".

As a feminist I am all for dismantling the gender binary. Nobody conforms to stereotypes of masculinity and femininity perfectly. These gendered boxes are restrictive and they enforce a social hierarchy that disadvantages females. This is why feminists see gender as means by which women are oppressed.

Women can try to identify as men in order to escape oppression. They can take testosterone, remove their breasts and uteruses, change their names and pronouns and even get certificates that say they are legally male. But they still won't be able to dominate men the way males, even those who identify as women, can physically overpower females.

Therefore, to say that women are oppressed due to some hypothesised inner identity of womanhood would require any analysis of sexism, misogyny and male violence to become uncoupled from the material reality, whereby women's oppression is, and has always been, linked to them being biologically female in a male-supremacist world.

As far as science is concerned, I always like to keep an open mind so I welcome more research into the transgender phenomenon. So far it seems that we are dealing with a pseudoscientific set of ideas which relies on misuse of language to justify a transgression of laws and existing social norms, rather than some groundbreaking new science that has turned our understanding of what it means to be male or female on its head.

Why is resisting certain policies related to gender identity so important to you?

I think it is important to resist any pseudoscience, especially if it seeks to influence medical treatment. As doctors we have the responsibility to be truthful and to first do no harm. Considering that sex can't be changed, and that masculinising females and feminising males with drugs and surgeries has no evidence to support it, whilst these interventions have risks (Madsen et al 2021) and some reported experiences of significant harm (Newgent 2021), then why are we offering these treatments in the first place?

Statistics also indicate that males who identify as women

retain male-pattern criminality (Dhejne 2011). If we change policy to segregate spaces such as prisons, healthcare, domestic violence shelters, toilets and sports, based on gender identity, rather than biological sex, we are introducing males into women's single-sex spaces, which increases the risk of harm. So I think we need to be highly sceptical of any practice that gives primacy to beliefs over observable facts, as this constitutes a departure from evidence-based policies into faith and peer-pressure driven decisions.

What is your view on the medical profession's general relationship to the concept of gender identity?

In medicine "masculine" and "feminine" have biological connotations. For example, exposure of a foetus to testosterone is said to "masculinise" them, and in the field of gender reassignment, we talk about masculinising females and feminising males to make them look like the opposite sex.

This is quite different from the social constructs of masculinity and femininity, which vary across cultures and time.

I think that these two meanings got conflated in the practice of gender reassignment, and this conflation is now spreading to other areas of medicine under the guise of "equality, diversity and inclusiveness."

Throughout history, males who were deemed to be insufficiently masculine were speculated to have a "feminine essence." Medicine later described this essence as "a woman trapped in a man's body", and attempted to "free it" with hormone blockers, cross-sex hormones and surgeries. Now, this essence is known as a "female gender identity" and scientists are trying to capture it with brain scans. I suspect that the reason why it hasn't been captured yet is because this "essence" is just a projection of society's discomfort with gender non-conformity.

What is the problem if we replace the category of sex with gender identity in medicine?

Biological sex is the most fundamental piece of information clinicians need in order to deliver safe and effective medical care. Male/female sex differences impact everything, from the likely diagnosis and lab reference ranges, to reactions to medication, choice of treatment, dosage and prognosis.

Despite this, the General Medical Council (GMC) has issued guidance (GMC, no date (1)) that asks doctors to "respect patient's request to change sex on their medical records." This process, which is facilitated by doctor's surgeries and Primary Care Support England (PCSE), involves issuing new NHS numbers with opposite sex markers and it removes all references to a patient's true biological sex (referred to as "previous gender identity") from the new record (LGBT Foundation 2020). According to the GMC, it is also "unlawful to disclose a patient's gender history without their consent."

Patients who decide to take advantage of these new rules risk not receiving invitations for sex-appropriate screening (Public Health England 2019) they can be misdiagnosed (Marchione 2019), and even denied appropriate medical treatment (Whitley et al 2017).

These new rules also restrict clinicians' autonomy to truthfully record and communicate relevant information pertaining to a patient's biological sex. All this seriously jeopardises healthcare of the very patient population these gender-identity-driven policies are meant to be benefitting.

Healthcare, of course, exists in a broader social context. For example, there's currently a push to use "gender neutral" language, so women are being referred to as "pregnant people," "menstruators" and "cervix-havers," however there are no corresponding descriptions such as "impregnators," "ejaculators" or "prostate-havers." Males are still referred to as "men," regardless of their gender identity.

Women are already underrepresented in clinical trials (Liu et al 2016). Their pain is taken less seriously, and due to atypical patterns in relation to males, their diagnoses such as a heart attack, can be delayed or missed, all of which affects long-term health outcomes. Replacing sex with gender identity in medicine would make sex-based research very difficult.

As many as one in four women is a survivor of male sexual violence, and in a medical setting, where we are all vulnerable, many women require access to single-sex spaces and same-sex healthcare providers in order to feel safe. When the GMC allowed doctors to self-identify as the opposite sex (GMC, no date (2)) on their professional register they made it very difficult for female patients to challenge male doctors who identify as women. In practice, patients who find themselves in this situation report being labelled "transphobic" and "difficult" when they complain. Many were worried that they would be refused medical care if they didn't keep quiet.

Abuse of females in a medical setting manifests in many different ways, from misogyny-driven medical scandals (Khaleeli 2014) and obstetric abuses (Deutsche Welle 2019) to sexual abuse of female patients by both male practitioners and male patients.

Replacing sex with gender identity in healthcare not only removes the protections women's sex-based rights give all females, it puts us in an impossible position where we can no longer use sex-based language to analyse and address the root causes of violence committed against us.

Many might assume that doctors are not susceptible to cultural or political influences. However, your work uncovers that parts of the medical establishment may have been persuaded to abandon some of their usual principles. Could you briefly outline some of what you discovered in your research on medical institutions and gender identity policies?

Replacing biological sex with gender identity in healthcare is a fundamental departure from the mainstream scientific understanding of human biology. Therefore such policies should have been a result of prolonged debate among clinicians. However, looking at the situation in the UK (la scapigliata 2021), policies that allow for the mis-sexing of patients and clinicians appear to have been imposed from above, by institutions who have signed up for various "equality, diversity and inclusiveness" schemes run by organisations such as Stonewall UK.

In some cases there is no electronic or paper trail to show us how these policies were developed and approved. Typically, no impact assessment was done to see how they would affect other protected characteristics, such as sex, disability, age, religion etc. Women are not routinely consulted. Instead, transactivists are seen as the sole stakeholders and allowed to influence administrators and small committees to make unilateral, belief-driven decisions.

Whenever I approached medical institutions, or their representatives, with concerns that women's sex-based rights were being breached by these new policies, I got stock replies that dismissed my concerns. The few colleagues who openly campaigned for gender self-identification would simply claim that "transwomen are women," call me a "transphobe" and refuse to engage further.

To what extent do you believe most doctors know what is going on?

I think doctors are increasingly aware of what is happening but they are under huge pressure due to the current public health crisis, the stressful nature of the job, as well as chronic understaffing and underfunding. Our institutions have implemented policies that would see you accused of bigotry and question your fitness to practice if you stated, quite correctly, that males aren't women. Most doctors' livelihood depends on not falling foul of these frameworks.

I receive confidential messages from colleagues and medical students all the time. They tell me they are afraid of being falsely accused of transphobia and face discrimination and bullying in their place of work/study if they openly question these policies. My feeling is that, the vast majority of healthcare professionals are concerned with the lack of evidence. They can see the many ways in which replacing sex with gender identity compromises patient healthcare and safety. However, the culture of dismissal and bullying has quashed all dissent, and this is being used by transactivists to claim that the medical profession fully endorses biology-denialism..

Why do you think some respected medical

organisations have been vulnerable to these influences?

Institutional capture was carried out quite systematically, using various tactics outlined in Denton's report titled "Only Adults? Good Practices in Legal Gender Recognition For Youth" (Dentons 2019), such as avoiding debate, tying gender identity proposals to less controversial policy suggestions (such as reforms to support LGB rights) and using youthful voices to portray these changes as "progressive." This has worked equally well at the GMC, British Medical Association (BMA), Care Quality Commission (CQC) and Royal Colleges as well as the Crown Prosecution Service (CPS), prison service and women's aid sector.

Clawing back from this will be difficult, because the gender identity lobby has had free reign for over a decade and now our institutions are riddled with policies made "in advance of the law". This makes lawful single-sex provisions all but impossible to enforce. Furthermore, free speech is under threat with increasingly Orwellian "hate crime" legislation and policing. However, with several Judicial Reviews under way that seek to examine the lawfulness of these policies, and their effect on individual service users, as well as growing public opposition, I am hopeful.

What are the duties of a doctor to their patients (especially women and girls) when it comes to understanding sex-based rights? For example, what would you see as the responsibilities of a medic who was born male but identifies as a woman when

seeking consent from a female patient to perform a breast examination?

Humans are sexually dimorphic, and we have evolved to instinctively recognise each other's biological sex. This instant recognition least relies on clothes, make-up, hair length or mannerisms. Our brains can be alerted to true biological sex by facial structure, voice, shoulder width, size of hands and feet, gait, scent, and as soon as any inconsistency is noted, the disguise no longer works. This is why even with the best cosmetic, surgical and hormonal interventions, transgender individuals rarely completely "pass" as the opposite sex, and this is especially true for males who identify as women.

Furthermore, sex recognition is context-dependent. We don't pay as much attention to the biological sex of people we casually pass on the street or interact with online, as we do in situations where we are vulnerable, such as being alone in a women's toilet or receiving a breast examination. .

This is why it's problematic that some male clinicians who identify as women report they might feel validated when female patients decline chaperones (Kamaruddin 2017). The imbalance of power between doctor and patient makes it unlikely the patient would challenge the doctor, and the apparent lack of insight about this is worrying.

Should a medic's sex be explicitly disclosed to the patient? Does such information impact a woman's ability to make an informed choice? Do you believe there are any conflicting rights for professionals to try to keep those details private?

I see biological sex as self-evident and gender identity as equivalent to any other belief system a doctor might hold, such as religion or membership in a political party. Belief systems, just like sexual orientation and other private information that isn't immediately apparent, don't need to be disclosed as long as they aren't negatively impacting treatment. As biological sex is obvious, it cannot constitute private information and it should be stated correctly.

If a female patient can recognise that a doctor is male despite his documents stating otherwise, but due to various policies she is not allowed to challenge him or demand a female practitioner without being accused of "transphobia", then she is being gaslit when she is in need of medical care and that is unacceptable.

Transactivists try to liken single-sex spaces and services to racial segregation or discrimination based on sexual orientation, but that is a false equivalence. Men being violent toward women is a well-documented problem in our society. We have no evidence that people of certain races or sexual orientations are more dangerous than others. Therefore, a woman requesting a female doctor is both reasonable and justified in light of male-pattern violence, while discrimination against a lesbian or a Black doctor would clearly be wrong.

Speaking both as a female patient and a survivor of male violence, any male doctor who disregards my concerns over this is automatically unsafe. The burden of proof needs to be on these doctors to demonstrate that they can put their belief systems aside, and focus on delivering safe and effective care to all patients, including women. That would mean a promise not to lie about their biological sex, declaring their biological sex correctly on all documents and respecting women's single-sex spaces and boundaries..

Yours seems one of few voices of dissent from the medical profession. Why do you think this is?

When I first became aware of these issues, the only perspectives I could find were either medical or feminist, so I thought I could contribute by combining the two. Male violence was already rife online, so I chose the nickname "la scapigliata", which means "head of a woman", to symbolise my free thoughts, spoken with no fear of death and rape threats, cyber stalking and other types of intimidation men are engaging in to silence women. I had hoped things would improve and that, eventually, I would be able to write under my own name, but unfortunately the violence toward women and feminists has since escalated.

In medicine there's also a risk of appearing "biased" if one should advocate for women's sex-based rights, even though the profession regards the male body and male authority as a default, which in practice means that male interests are heavily prioritised. This medical sexism is so deeply entrenched, that even in healthcare settings, the very concept of male-free spaces and women being allowed to say "No" to males is still very controversial.

How has writing about this issue affected you?

Since I started writing about the cognitive and policy capture of the medical profession by the concept of gender identity, the stakes have risen and I would lie if I said that this hasn't taken a toll on me. Seeing how far our profession has departed from "first, do no harm" and evidence-based decision making, and having to conduct this debate in an extremely hostile environment, is very stressful.

This work has also taken a lot of time and energy away from

other projects. I have not received any payment for the countless hours of intellectual work I have undertaken, and I am not the only one. Women and men from all walks of life - lawyers, teachers, doctors, counsellors, parents, sports coaches - are doing the work our institutions have failed to do. We are identifying pitfalls, analysing and challenging gender identity policies in the media, with the institutions directly and through the courts, and at best, we can hope that some of these dangerous policies are reluctantly withdrawn with no reflection or apology. It feels daunting.

What is your advice for any other concerned doctors or medical students, particularly those who might be afraid of engaging with this subject?

Medical students need to learn how to be safe and competent doctors, a task that is that much harder in an environment where language and science are being compromised by the introduction of thought crimes and pseudoscience. My advice to them is to focus on evidence-based information and on learning to critically appraise research, because these skills will be most helpful in separating scientific fact from belief-based assertions.

Doctors have a job to do and families to feed, so don't do anything that would jeopardise that. But do write to your College, Trust, BMA, GMC, MP, the papers, whenever you feel able, and do what you can to avoid mis-sexing patients in medical notes. Connect with like-minded colleagues at work and spend more time with your children, to make sure they aren't being groomed to uncritically accept unscientific ideas around gender identity. Go to the Mumsnet feminist sub-forum and gender-critical Twitter. Look at the work of the Society for Evidence Based Gender Medicine (SEGM), Fair Play for

Women and Transgender Trend. Soon, UK doctors will have their own group and website that will offer an alternative to the affirmation-only approach. The tide is turning so come and join us if and when you can.

What are your hopes for the future? Any bright spots on the horizon?

One huge bright spot is that, if we can expose the false equivalencies between transgender and intersex, then awareness of DSDs, how people are affected by them and all the medical harms inflicted on this patient population may become more mainstream knowledge. This will help this marginalised patient population receive better medical care and experience less social stigma.

Another benefit is that gender identity policies have exposed weaknesses in systems designed to provide child safeguarding and sex-based protections for women. We cannot fix what we don't know is broken, so this gives us an opportunity to improve.

Finally, I think these policies of gender identity have put gender stereotypes under a magnifying glass and I hope we will emerge from this with far greater tolerance toward gender non-conformity. Our culture is still sexually exploitative of women, as well as homophobic, and this set of ideas around gender identity amplifies these prejudices to an absurd degree. It is my hope that, going forward, we can move away from gender stereotyping. This will improve the health and wellbeing of everyone, including people who identify as transgender..

Where can women find your work, and what can they do to support you?

You can find me on twitter as @lascapigliata8 and on my blog www.lascapigliata.com. I have been fortunate enough to have received a lot of support from feminists, colleagues and members of public. There is safety in numbers, so the best way to support us is to join us.

Bibliography

FiLiA (2021). A Feminist Doctor on Gender Identity Policies, Institutional Capture and Medicine. https://www.filia.org.uk/latest-news/2021/3/24/a-feminist-doctor-on-gender-identity-policies-institutional-capture-and-medicine

Dhejne, C. Lichtenstein, P. Boman, M. Johansson, A.L.V. Långström, N. Landén, M. (2011). Long-Term Follow-Up of Transsexual Persons Undergoing Sex Reassignment Surgery: Cohort Study in Sweden. PLoS ONE 6(2): e16885. https://doi.org/10.1371/journal.pone.0016885

Evans, M. (2021). Freedom to think: The need for thorough assessment and treatment of gender dysphoric children. BJPsych Bulletin, 45(5), 285-290. doi:10.1192/bjb.2020.72 https://www.cambridge.org/core/journals/bjpsych-bulletin/article/freedom-to-think-the-need-for-thorough-assessment-and-treatment-of-gender-dysphoric-children/F4B7F5CAFC0D0BE9FF3C7886BA6E904B

Zucker, K. (2015). (PDF) The DSM-5 Diagnostic Criteria for Gender Dysphoria. ResearchGate. https://link.springer.com/chapter/10.1007/978-88-470-5696-1_4

Hilton, E. (2018). Here follows some data from karyotype studies in newborns. These are cohort studies, systematically recording birth sex, sex chromosome conformation and any notable phenotype in sequential births at maternity units over extended periods of time. https://mobile.twitter.com/FondOfBeetles/status/1111352888385769472

Sax, L. (2002). How Common Is Intersex? A Response to Anne Fausto-Sterling. The Journal of Sex Research, 39(3), 174–178. https://www.leonardsax.com/how-common-is-intersex-a-response-to-anne-fausto-sterling/

Pang, K. C. Feldman, D. Oerter, R. and Telfer, M. (2018). Molecular Karyotyping in Children and Adolescents with Gender Dysphoria. Transgender Health, Dec 2018, 147-153. http://doi.org/10.1089/trgh.2017.0051

Griffin, L. Clyde, K. Byng, R. & Bewley, S. (2021). Sex, gender and gender identity: A re-evaluation of the evidence. BJPsych Bulletin, 45(5), 291-299. doi:10.1192/bjb.2020.73 https://www.cambridge.org/core/journals/bjpsych-bulletin/article/sex-gender-and-gender-identity-a-reevaluation-of-the-evidence/76A3DC54F3BD91E8D631B93397698B1A

Madsen, M. C. van Dijk, D. Wiepjes, C. M. Conemans, E. B. Thijs, A. &

Bibliography

den Heijer, M. (2021). Erythrocytosis in a Large Cohort of Trans Men Using Testosterone: A Long-Term Follow-Up Study on Prevalence, Determinants, and Exposure Years. The Journal of clinical endocrinology and metabolism, 106(6), 1710–1717. https://pubmed.ncbi.nlm.nih.gov/33599731/

Newgent, S. (2021). We need balance when it comes to gender dysphoric kids. I would know | Opinion. Newsweek. https://www.newsweek.com/we-need-balance-when-it-comes-gender-dysphoric-kids-i-would-know-opinion-1567277

GMC. (no date (1)). Trans healthcare. Gmc-uk.org. https://www.gmc-uk.org/ethical-guidance/ethical-hub/trans-healthcare#confidentiality-and-equality

LGBT Foundation. (2020). Changing a patient's name and gender marker. Weobleyandstauntonsurgeries.nhs.uk. https://www.weobleyandstauntonsurgeries.nhs.uk/website/M81018/files/Changing%20Your%20name%20and%20Gender%20with%20the%20NHS.pdf

Public Health England. (2019). Should trans men have cervical screening tests?. nhs.uk. https://www.nhs.uk/common-health-questions/sexual-health/should-trans-men-have-cervical-screening-tests/

Marchione, M. (2019). Nurse mistakes pregnant transgender man as obese. Then, the man births a stillborn baby. Eu.usatoday.com. https://eu.usatoday.com/story/news/health/2019/05/16/pregnant-transgender-man-births-stillborn-baby-hospital-missed-labor-signs/3692201002/

Whitley, C., Greene, D. (2017) Transgender Man Being Evaluated for a Kidney Transplant. Clinical Chemistry, Volume 63, Issue 11, 1 November 2017, Pages 1680–1683, https://doi.org/10.1373/clinchem.2016.268839 https://academic.oup.com/clinchem/article/63/11/1680/5612702

Liu, K. A., & Mager, N. A. (2016). Women's involvement in clinical trials: historical perspective and future implications. Pharmacy practice, 14(1), 708. https://doi.org/10.18549/PharmPract.2016.01.708

GMC. (no date (2)). Maintain your registration. Gmc-uk.org. https://www.gmc-uk.org/registration-and-licensing/managing-your-registration/information-for-doctors-on-the-register/maintain-your-registration

Khaleeli, H. (2014). Symphysiotomy – Ireland's brutal alternative to caesareans. theguardian.com. https://www.theguardian.com/lifeandstyle/2014/dec/12/symphysiotomy-irelands-brutal-alternative-to-caesareans

Deutsche Welle. (2019). Women around the world face widespread abuse during childbirth | DW | 25.11.2019. DW.COM. https://www.dw.com/en/

Bibliography

women-around-the-world-face-widespread-abuse-during-childbirth/a-51393868

la scapigliata. (2021). Investigation into the influence of gender ideology on medical institutions. https://lascapigliata.com/2021/01/07/investigation-into-the-influence-of-gender-ideology-on-medical-institutions/

Dentons. (2019). Only Adults? Good Practices in Legal Gender Recognition for Youth - A report on the current state of laws and NGO advocacy in eight countries in Europe, with a focus on rights of young people. Iglyo.com. https://www.iglyo.com/wp-content/uploads/2019/11/IGLYO_v3-1.pdf

Kamaruddin, K. (2017). What it's like to be a transgender patient and a GP. British Journal of General Practice 2017; 67 (660): 313. DOI: 10.3399/bjgp17X691433. https://bjgp.org/content/67/660/313

Acknowledgments

I would like to thank my dear friend Lorelei (@hatpinwoman) for her invaluable editorial advice and encouragement, and Mole at the Counter (@moleatthedoor) for creating such a beautiful book cover.

I am deeply grateful to radical feminists and other members of the growing "gender critical" community who selflessly shared their testimonies, knowledge, and expertise with me.

Most of all, I want to thank my husband for his unwavering love and support.

About the Author

Isidora Sanger is the nom-de-plume of Dr Maja Bowen, a retired medical doctor, also known as "la scapigliata" online. Since 2014, she's been writing about gender identity ideology and campaigning for women's sex-based rights. She believes policies and medical practices should be based on evidence, not ideology.

She lives in the UK with her family and a dog.

Printed in Great Britain
by Amazon